AF166844

Pelvic Floor Ultrasound

Lewis Chan • Vincent Tse
Stephanie The • Peter Stewart
Editors

Pelvic Floor Ultrasound

Principles, Applications and Case Studies

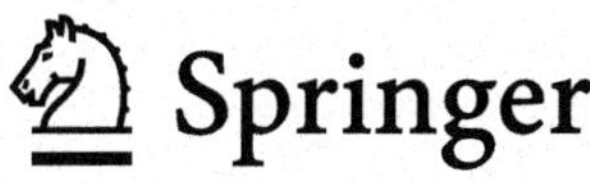

Springer

Editors
Lewis Chan
Department of Urology
Concord Repatriation General Hospital
Sydney, New South Wales, Australia

Vincent Tse
Department of Urology
Concord Repatriation General Hospital
Sydney, New South Wales, Australia

Stephanie The
Department of Women's
and Children's Health
Pelvic Floor Unit
Westmead Hospital
Sydney, New South Wales, Australia

Peter Stewart
Department of Colorectal Surgery
Concord Repatriation General Hospital
Sydney, New South Wales, Australia

ISBN 978-3-319-04309-8 ISBN 978-3-319-04310-4 (eBook)
DOI 10.1007/978-3-319-04310-4

Library of Congress Control Number: 2015932253

Springer Cham Heidelberg New York Dordrecht London

Printed on acid-free paper

Springer International Publishing AG Switzerland is part of Springer Science+Business Media
(www.springer.com)

Foreword

All you wanted to know about pelvic floor ultrasound….and more!

This very focused book on Pelvic Floor Ultrasound was designed with the clinician in mind. There is no doubt that the pelvic floor area crosses many health professionals, including urologists, gynecologists, colorectal surgeons and physical therapists to name a few. The field has expanded so much that female pelvic medicine and reconstructive surgery is now a new sub-specialty with its own certification process in the United States. Almost all experts in the area of FPMRS will need more than findings on clinical history and examination to better investigate and understand the key organs and pelvic structure beyond the confines of the vagina. Ultrasound is a safe technology, which is operator dependent both in terms of performance and interpretation. Trained eyes can see pelvic floor disorders that others won't. This book is the best available resource so far to take the novice and experts alike through the unique features of this important imaging modality. The authors have conducted workshops on pelvic floor imaging using ultrasound the world over. They are staunch advocates of the integration of this modality into our clinician practice.

The structure of this book is very simple, practical, and hands-on. The first chapters are dedicated to the principles of ultrasound and to ultrasound instrumentation. The ensuing chapters address practical aspects such as choosing your ultrasound equipment, setting up your ultrasound room, and clearing the accreditation processes. Next, the authors, with their broad expertise in urology, colorectal surgery and gynecology, take on the tasks of covering male and female voiding dysfunction, pelvic organ prolapse and fecal incontinence. Finally the book ends on a ninth chapter focusing on 3D ultrasound. Each chapter has a unique structure including case studies, practical tips presented in table format, and short video clips to illustrate real-time imaging findings.

As the result of the authors' expertise, teaching skills honed through years of giving courses on pelvic floor imaging, and daily incorporation of pelvic floor ultrasound in their clinical practice, the reader will find this book very approachable, extremely resourceful, and utterly relevant.

So here it is…pelvic ultrasound imaging at your fingertips! Yes, this book will convince you to incorporate this procedure in your practice. Yes, it will serve as an extension of what your fingers cannot touch or appreciate beyond the wall of the vagina. Yes, it will benefit your patients and make you better clinicians. Yes, it may change completely your diagnostic accuracy and likely will alter your management plans. At the very least, it will make you more appreciative of the enormous potentials of this safe, well-established, yet technically evolving technology. Enjoy your reading…and then get started!

Philippe Zimmern, MD, FACS
Professor, Department of Urology
Jane and John Justin Distinguished Chair in Urology,
University of Texas Southwestern Medical Center
Dallas, Texas, USA

Preface

Urinary incontinence, faecal incontinence and pelvic organ prolapse are significant health problems. Patients may come under the care of many different health professionals including urologists, gynaecologists, colorectal surgeons and physiotherapists.

There is increasing interest in using ultrasound for assessment of pelvic floor dysfunction, and clinicians are uniquely placed to utilize this dynamic form of imaging. The urologist, gynaecologist and colo-rectal surgeon with a good understanding of the structure and function of the pelvic organs can integrate the clinical presentation, functional studies (e.g. urodynamics/ anorectal physiology) with imaging to provide better assessment and care for the patient. Whilst ultrasound equipment is widely available around the world, many clinicians may not have access to structured training in the technique of pelvic floor imaging and interpretation of images in the context of pelvic floor dysfunction. This book is written for clinicians who wish to explore the technique which is really an extension of clinical examination of the patient. There are step-by-step guides to starting up in performing pelvic floor ultrasound and tricks of the trade 'tips' in how to obtain good images. We have included case studies of common conditions to illustrate the role of ultrasound in assisting the clinician to manage pelvic floor disorders and the benefits of incorporating ultrasound imaging into one's clinical practice. There is an introduction to the 3D ultrasound techniques for the interested clinician wishing to take advantage of this emerging modality which is of increasing relevance in the management of complex pelvic floor dysfunction.

Good quality images are key to allow accurate interpretation of imaging findings. The editors are indebted to Dr. Fulgham, the previous Chair of the American Urological Association Urologic Ultrasound Faculty, for contributing the introductory chapters on the basic principles of ultrasound and techniques for optimizing the ultrasound image which are the important pre-requisites to performing clinician-performed ultrasound.

We hope the contents of this book will encourage you and provide the basis for starting your journey in ultrasound of the pelvic floor!

Sydney, Australia
November 2014

Lewis Chan
Vincent Tse
Stephanie The
Peter Stewart

Contents

1 **The Physics and Technique of Ultrasound** 1
Pat F. Fulgham

2 **Machine Settings and Technique of Image Optimization** 25
Pat F. Fulgham

3 **Essentials for Setting Up Practice in Clinician Performed Ultrasound** 39
Lewis Chan

4 **Ultrasound Imaging in Assessment of the Male Patient with Voiding Dysfunction** 45
Lewis Chan, Tom Jarvis, Stuart Baptist, and Vincent Tse

5 **Pelvic Ultrasound in the Assessment of Female Voiding Dysfunction** 63
Lewis Chan

6 **Practical Application of Ultrasound in the Assessment of Pelvic Organ Prolapse** 77
Vincent Tse and Lewis Chan

7 **Ultrasound Imaging of Gynaecologic Organs** 87
Stephanie The

8 **Endoanal Ultrasound of Pelvic Floor** 109
Peter Stewart

9 **Principles and Applications of 3D Pelvic Floor Ultrasound** 125
Shelley O'Sullivan, Vincent Tse, Stephanie The, Lewis Chan, and Peter Stewart

Index 147

Contributors

Stuart Baptist BSc (Hons)Physio, RPT, APAM, CFA Sydney Sports and Orthopaedic Physiotherapy Group, Sydney, NSW, Australia

Lewis Chan MBBS(Hons), FRACS, DDU Department of Urology, Concord Repatriation General Hospital, Sydney, NSW, Australia

Pat F. Fulgham MD, DABU, FACS Department of Urology, Texas Health Presbyterian Hospital of Dallas, Dallas, TX, USA

Thomas R. Jarvis BSc(Med), MBBS(Hons), FRACS(Uro) Department of Urology, Prince of Wales Hospital, Randwick, NSW, Australia

Shelley O'Sullivan RDMS Ultrasound, Philips Healthcare Australia, North Ryde, NSW, Australia

Peter Stewart MBBS, FRACS Department of Colo-Rectal Surgery, Concord Repatriation General Hospital, Sydney, Australia

Stephanie The MBBS, FRANZCOG, DDU, COGU Department of Women's and Children's Health, Pelvic Floor Unit, Westmead Hospital, Sydney, NSW, Australia

Vincent Tse MBBS, MS, FRACS Department of Urology, Concord Repatriation General Hospital, Sydney, NSW, Australia

Chapter 1
The Physics and Technique of Ultrasound

Pat F. Fulgham

Ultrasound performed and interpreted by the clinician combines knowledge of the anatomy and disease processes with technical expertise to produce images of superior quality which answer a specific clinical question. An understanding of the physical principles of ultrasound, proper probe selection and machine settings is critical to obtaining high quality diagnostic images. This chapter will describe the physical principles of ultrasound along with an explanation for how to adjust machine settings to correct for common ultrasound artifacts.

Physics of Ultrasound

The images generated by ultrasound are created by the interaction between the mechanical ultrasound waves and human tissue. Ultrasound requires a conducting medium (ultrasound gel) and a physical medium such as tissue or fluid. The ultrasound waves are transmitted into the body by the transducer and then reflected back to the transducer at frequent intervals producing a real-time image. The transducer acts as both a sender and a receiver.

The sound waves are generated by electrical impulses which are converted to mechanical sound waves via the piezoelectric effect. The piezoelectric effect [1] occurs when alternating current is applied to a crystal containing dipoles. Areas of charge within a piezoelectric element are distributed in patterns which yield a "net" positive and negative orientation. When alternating charge is applied to both faces of the element, a relative contraction or elongation of the charged areas occurs, resulting in a mechanical expansion and then a contraction of the element (Fig. 1.1).

P.F. Fulgham, MD, DABU, FACS
Department of Urology, Texas Health Presbyterian Hospital of Dallas,
8210 Walnut Hill Suite 014, Dallas, TX 75231, USA
e-mail: pfulgham@airmail.net

L. Chan et al. (eds.), *Pelvic Floor Ultrasound: Principles, Applications and Case Studies*, DOI 10.1007/978-3-319-04310-4_1

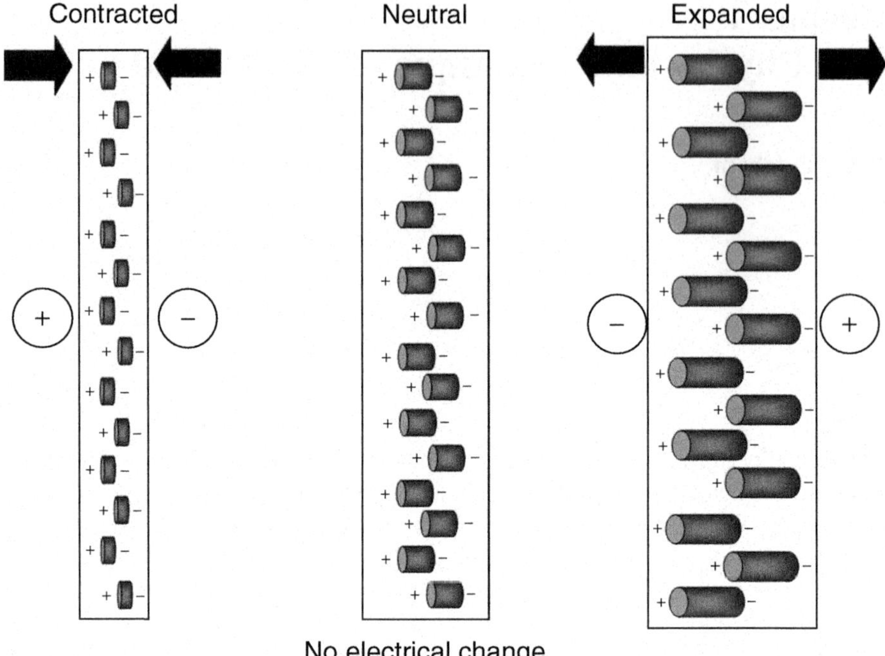

Fig. 1.1 Piezoelectric effect. Areas of "net" charge within a crystal expand or contract when current is applied to the surface, creating a mechanical wave. When the returning wave strikes the crystal an electrical current is generated

This results in a mechanical wave which is transmitted into the patient. These ultrasound waves are longitudinal waves which produce compression and rarefaction of tissue in the direction of the wave (Fig. 1.2).

Reflected mechanical sound waves are received by the transducer and converted back into electrical energy via the piezoelectric effect. The electrical energy is interpreted via software within the ultrasound instrument to generate an image which is displayed upon the monitor.

This compression and rarefaction of molecules can be represented graphically as a sine wave (Fig. 1.3) which alternates between a positive and negative deflection from the baseline. The wavelength is the distance between one peak of the wave and the next peak. A cycle is the complete path of the wave. One cycle per second is known as 1 Hz (Hertz). The maximal excursion of the wave in the positive or negative direction from the baseline is the amplitude of the wave. The time it takes for one complete cycle of the wave is known as the period. The amplitude of the wave is a function of the acoustical power used to generate the mechanical compression wave and the medium through which it is transmitted.

For most modes of ultrasound, the transducer emits a limited number of wave cycles (usually two to four) called a pulse. The frequency of the two to four wave cycles, called the pulse repetition frequency, is usually less than 2 KHz. The transducer

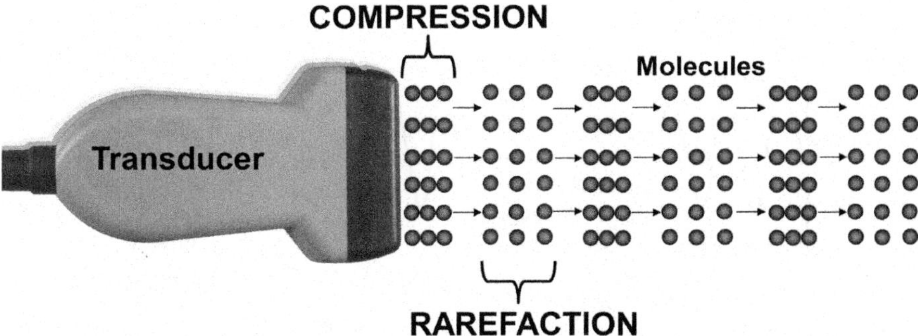

Fig. 1.2 Longitudinal waves are created by the expansion and contraction of piezoelectric crystals within the transducer. These waves are created when an alternating current is applied to the crystals which create compression and rarefaction of molecules in the body

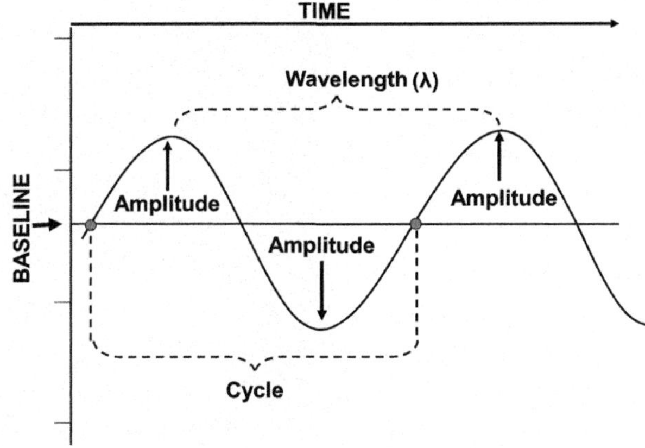

Fig. 1.3 Sine wave: when referring to a sine wave a cycle represents the path of the wave from above the baseline then below the baseline and back to the baseline

is then "silent" as it awaits the return of the reflected waves from within the body (Fig. 1.4). The transducer serves as a receiver more than 99 % of the time.

The pulse repetition frequency (PRF) is the number of pulses being sent out per unit time. By timing the pulse from transmission to reception it is possible to calculate the distance from the transducer to the object reflecting the wave. This is known as ultrasound ranging (Fig. 1.5). This sequence is known as pulsed-wave ultrasound.

Ultrasound ranging depends on assumptions about the average velocity of ultrasound in human tissue to locate reflectors in the ultrasound field. The elapsed time from pulse transmission to reception of the same pulse by the transducer allows for determining the location of a reflector in the ultrasound field.

The amplitude of the returning waves determines the brightness of the pixel assigned to the reflector in an ultrasound image. The greater the amplitude of the returning wave the brighter the pixel assigned. Thus, an ultrasound unit produces an "image" by first causing a transducer to emit a series of ultrasound waves at specific frequencies and intervals and then interpreting the returning echoes for duration of

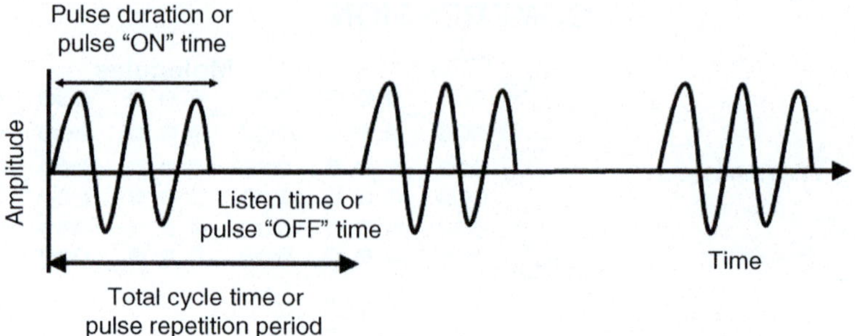

Fig. 1.4 The pulsed-wave ultrasound mode depends on an emitted pulse of 2–4 wave cycles followed by a period of "silence" as the transducer awaits the return of the emitted pulse

Fig. 1.5 Demonstrates ultrasound ranging. The elapsed time from the transducer (*A*) to a bladder tumor (*B*) is 0.045 ms. The total time it takes to travel back to the transducer (*C*) is 0.09 ms

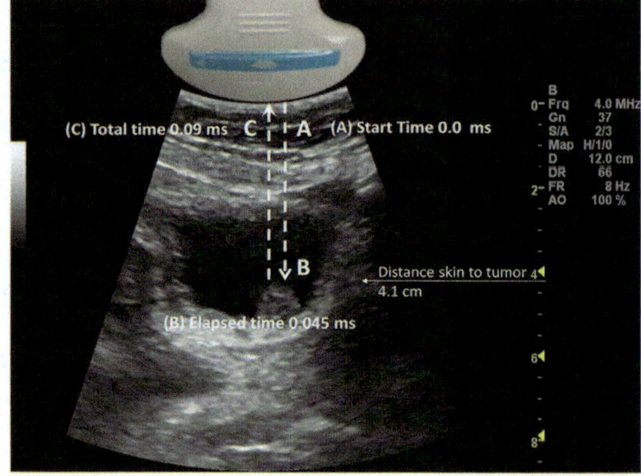

transit and amplitude. This "image" is rapidly refreshed on a monitor to give the impression of continuous motion. Frame refresh rates are typically 12–30/s. The sequence of events depicted in Fig. 1.6 is the basis for all "scanned" modes of ultrasound including the familiar gray-scale ultrasound.

Frequency and wavelength affect the velocity with which sound travels through tissue. The velocity of sound in tissue is constant; therefore, changing the frequency will change the wavelength and influence the depth of penetration.

The velocity with which a sound wave travels through tissue is a product of its frequency and its wavelength. The velocity of sound in a given tissue is constant. Therefore, as the frequency of the sound wave changes the wavelength must also change. The average velocity of sound in human tissues is 1,540 m/s. Wavelength and frequency vary in an inverse relationship. Velocity equals frequency times wavelength. As the frequency diminishes from 10 to 1 MHz the wavelength increases from 0.15 to 1.5 mm. This has important consequences for the choice of transducer depending on the indication for imaging.

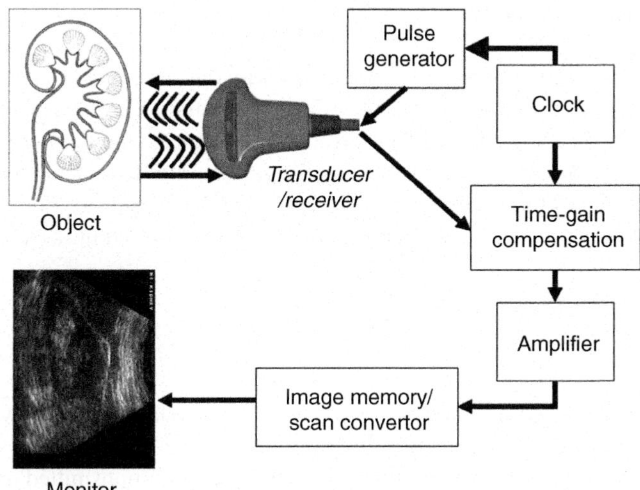

Fig. 1.6 Schematic depiction of the sequence of image production by an ultrasound device

Common Ultrasound Interactions with Human Tissue

Ultrasound waves are altered in a variety of ways as they interact with human tissue. There may be loss of energy, change in direction or a change in frequency. In order to maximize image quality and correctly interpret the images the sonographer must understand these interactions.

Attenuation

Sound waves lose energy as they interact with tissue and fluid within the body [2]. This interaction is called attenuation. Attenuation is measured in dB/cm/MHz. The greater is the attenuation, the more energy is lost as the soundwave passes through the tissue. The amount of attenuation that may occur varies by specific tissues. For example, the kidney has an attenuation of 1.0 and muscle an attenuation of 3.3. Therefore, sound waves will lose more energy as they pass through muscle.

The three most important mechanisms of attenuation are absorption, reflection and scattering. Absorption occurs when the mechanical kinetic energy of a sound wave is converted to heat within the tissue. Absorption is dependent on the frequency of the sound wave and the characteristics of the attenuating tissue. Higher frequency waves are more rapidly attenuated by absorption than lower frequency waves.

Correcting for Attenuation

Since sound waves are progressively attenuated with distance traveled, deep structures in the body (for example kidney) are more difficult to image. Compensation for loss of acoustic energy by attenuation can be accomplished by selecting a lower frequency or by increasing the acoustic power. Adjusting the gain settings to increase the sensitivity of the transducer to the returning sound waves and will result in a brighter image, however, it will not increase the effective energy of the reflected ultrasound wave.

Refraction

Refraction occurs when a sound wave encounters an interface between two tissues of differing impedance and at any angle other than 90°. When a wave strikes an interface at an angle a portion of the wave is reflected and a portion is transmitted into the adjacent tissue. The transmitted wave is refracted, which results in a loss of some information because the wave is not completely reflected back to the transducer (Fig. 1.7).

There are also potential errors in registration of object location because of the refraction of the wave.

Correcting for Refraction

Refraction may be minimized by altering the angle of insonation to make it as close to 90° as feasible.

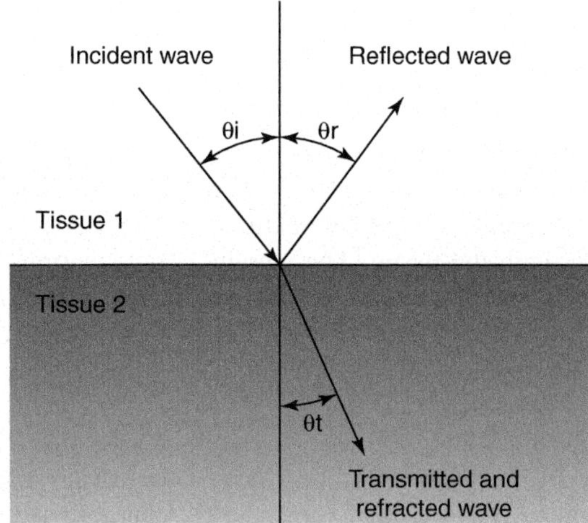

Fig. 1.7 When a wave strikes the interface between two tissues of differing impedance, the wave is usually partially reflected and partially transmitted with refraction. A portion of the wave is reflected (θR) at an angle equal to the angle of insonation (θi), a portion of the wave is transmitted at a refracted (θt) angle into the second tissue

Reflection

Reflection which occurs when a sound wave strikes an object with a large flat surface is called a *specular reflection*. Specular reflection may occur, for example, when sound waves strike the bladder wall during pelvic ultrasound.

Diffuse reflection occurs when an object is small or irregular resulting in a scattering pattern or "speckle effect". This type of reflection may often be seen with ultrasound of the uterus or testis (Fig. 1.8).

Correcting for Reflection

Recognizing reflection as a normal occurrence with ultrasound as opposed to a pathological abnormality of tissue is important. This is a physical property of ultrasound waves and there are no machine settings to correct for reflection. When reflection impedes the interpretation of some portion of the ultrasound field, it can be mitigated by changing the angle of insonation.

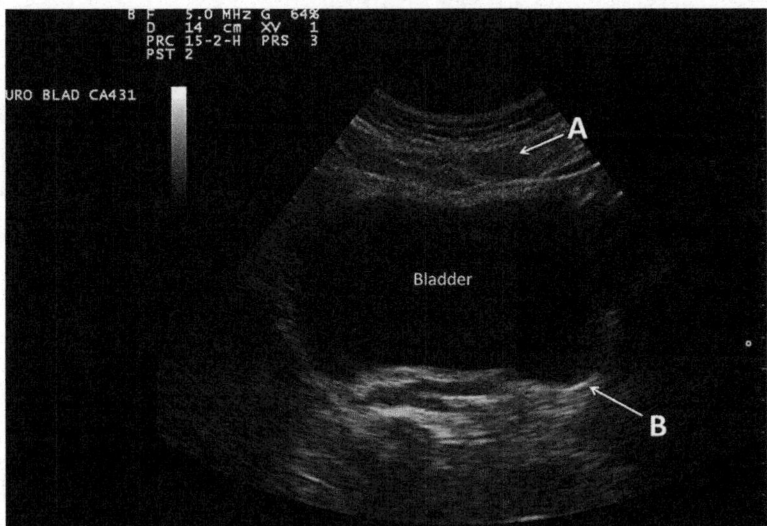

Fig. 1.8 In this transverse image of the bladder, the rectus abdominis muscle (*A*) is a diffuse reflector. Note the speculated or finely granular nature of the muscle. The bladder wall (*B*) serves as a specular reflector. A specular reflector reflects sound waves at an angle equal to the incident angle without producing a pattern of interference caused by scattering

Table 1.1 Impedance of tissue

Tissue	Density (kg/m^3)	Impedance
Air and other gases	1.2	0.0004
Fat tissue	952	1.38
Water and other clear liquids	1,000	1.48
Kidney (average of soft tissue)	1,060	1.63
Liver	1,060	1.64
Muscle	1,080	1.70
Bone and other calcified objects	1,912	7.8

Adapted from *Diagnostic Ultrasound*, 3rd ed, vol. 1
Impedance (Z) is a product of tissue density (p) and the velocity of that tissue (c). Impedance is defined by the formula: Z(Rayles) = p(kg/m^3) × c(m/s)

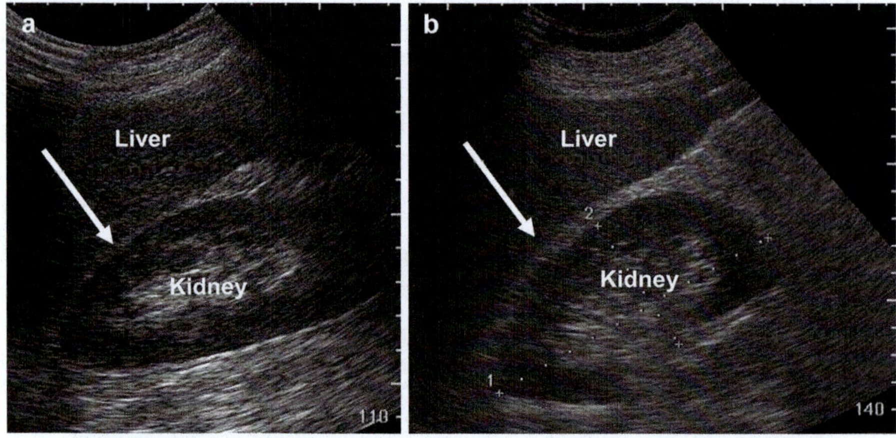

Fig. 1.9 Image (**a**) demonstrates that when kidney and liver are directly adjacent to each other it is difficult to appreciate the boundary between the capsules of the kidney and liver (*arrow*). Image (**b**) demonstrates that when fat, which has significantly lower impedance (*arrow*) is interposed it is far easier to appreciate the boundary between liver capsule and fat

Impedance

Impedance occurs when a certain amount of energy is reflected at the interface between tissues of differing tissue density. The amount of energy reflected increases when there is a greater difference between the tissue. For example, there is very little difference in impedance between kidney (1.63) and liver (1.64) so it is difficult to distinguish between these two organs unless there is a layer of fat around the kidney which has a lower impedance factor of 1.38 (Table 1.1).

Fat has a sufficient impedance difference from both kidney and liver that the borders of the two organs can be distinguished by virtue of the intervening fat (Fig. 1.9).

If the impedance differences between tissues are very high, complete reflection of sound waves may occur, resulting in acoustic shadowing (Fig. 1.10).

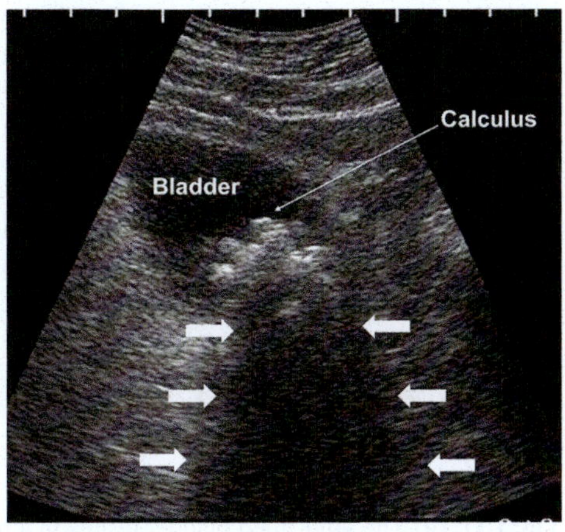

Fig. 1.10 In the urinary bladder, reflection of sound waves is the result of large impedance differences between urine and the bladder calculus (*thin arrow*). Acoustic shadowing results from nearly complete reflection of sound waves (area between the *thick arrows*)

Correcting for Impedance

There are no machine settings to correct for impedance. Imaging the patient from different angles to avoid the interface with large impedance differences may be helpful. In the case of a patient with bladder stones, having the patient physically turn or rotate will cause the stones to move, confirm the presence of the mobile stones and allow imaging of different parts of the bladder.

Common Artifacts

Sound waves are emitted from the ultrasound transducer with a known amplitude, direction, and frequency. However, interactions with tissues in the body result in alterations of these parameters. Because of the physical properties of ultrasound and the assumption by software algorithms in the ultrasound machine that returning sound waves have undergone alterations according to expected physical principles such as attenuation with distance, images are sometimes produced which do not accurately reflect the underlying anatomy. These are known as artifacts. Knowing the most common artifacts in ultrasound and how to correct for them is important when performing and interpreting ultrasound

Increased Through-Transmission

When sound waves pass through tissue that has less attenuation than surrounding tissue "increased through-transmission" will result. For example, the area distal to a fluid-filled bladder will appear brighter than surrounding histologically identical tissue. This hyperechogenicity may obscure structures within the area of increased through-transmission (Fig. 1.11).

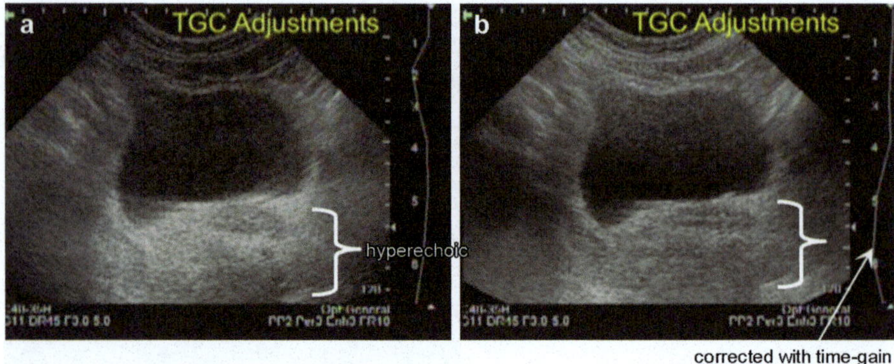

Fig. 1.11 (**a**) The fluid-filled bladder results in a region of decreased attenuation which produces a hyperechoic appearance in the tissue posterior to the urinary bladder (*bracket*). (**b**) This artifact called "increased thru-transmission" (*bracket*) can be corrected by decreasing the TGC curve in this region (*arrow*)

Correcting for Increased Through-Transmission

This artifact can be overcome by changing the angle of insonation or adjusting the time-gain compensation (TGC) (Fig. 1.11b). Reducing the gain level in the area distal to the bladder will decrease the brightness. The relative echogenicity of tissues known to be structurally or histologically identical should be consistent from the top of the image to the bottom.

Acoustic Shadowing

If there is significant attenuation of sound waves, acoustic shadowing may occur. This may occur at the interface between tissues of different impedance and will result in an anechoic or hyperechoic shadow. Information about the region distal to the interface will be lost or diminished.

Correcting for Acoustic Shadowing

The problems with acoustic shadowing are most appropriately overcome by changing the angle of insonation or changing the position of the target organ. This can be done by turning the patient (e.g. turning a patient on their side to gain access to the kidney lateral to the intestine) or by compression of the abdomen with the probe to move bowel gas aside. In pelvic scanning a roll can be placed beneath the buttock to improve the angle of insonation to the prostate posterior to the pubic bone (Fig. 1.12).

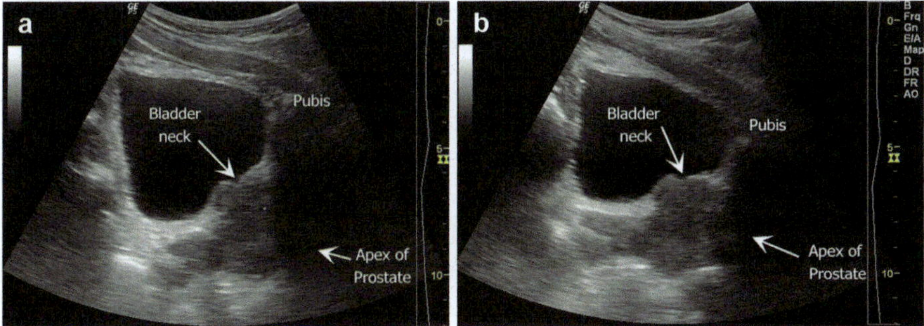

Fig. 1.12 (**a**) In this sagittal, transabdominal image of the bladder and prostate, there is a shadow distal to the pubis obscuring the apex of the prostate (*arrow*). (**b**) In this image, a roll has been placed under the patient's buttocks (*arrow*) to lift this pelvis enabling the probe to be angled thus displaying more of the apex of the prostate

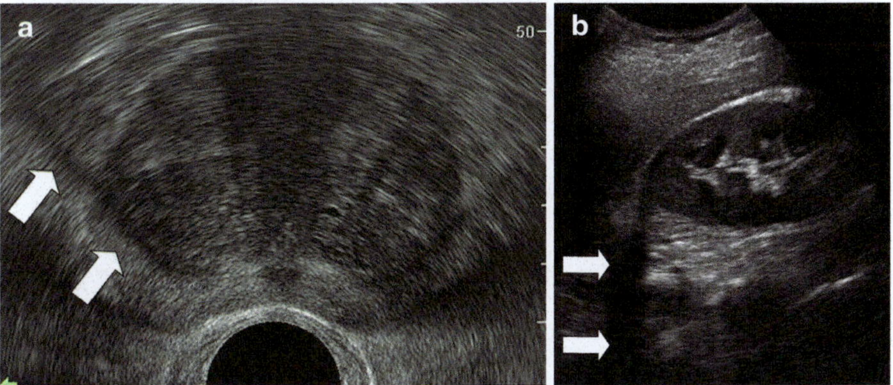

Fig. 1.13 (**a**) Edging artifact seen in this transverse image of the prostate is the result of the lack of reflection of the sound wave from the curved lateral surface of the transition zone (*thick arrows*). (**b**) Edging artifact caused by the rounded upper pole of the kidney (*thick arrows*)

Edging Artifact

Edging artifact occurs when an ultrasound wave strikes a curved surface. The sound wave is refracted at the critical angle of insonation resulting in a shadow and a loss of information distal to the interface (Fig. 1.13).

Correcting for Edging Artifact

Edging artifact is usually corrected by changing the angle of insonation.

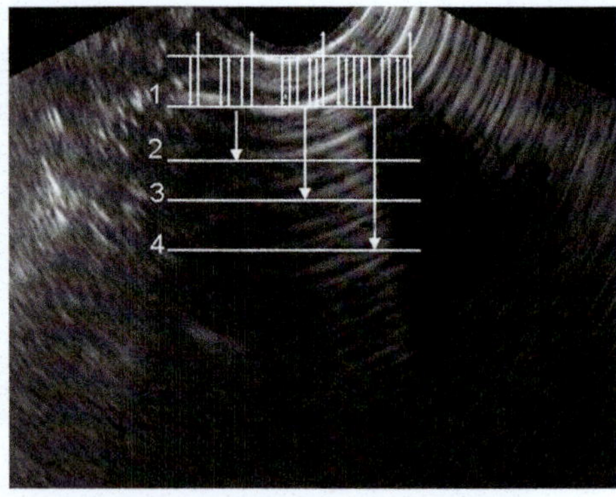

Fig. 1.14 A reverberation artifact occurs when a sound wave is repeatedly reflected between two interfaces. The resultant echo pattern is a collection of artifactual hyperechoic echoes distal to the structure with progressive attenuation of the sound wave

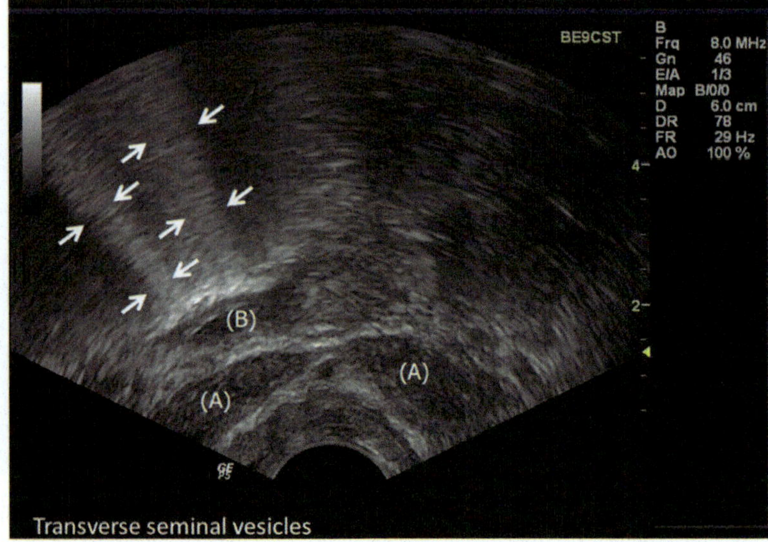

Fig. 1.15 In this transverse image of the seminal vesicles (*A*), a loop of small bowel (*B*) containing gas and fluid creates an example of a reverberation artifact (*arrows*)

Reverberation Artifact

Reverberation artifact occurs when there are large differences in impedance between two adjacent structures or surfaces resulting in two strong reflective interfaces. The sound wave reverberates between the two interfaces. As the sound wave is successively reflected there is ongoing attenuation with each reverberation. This produces echoes that are equally spaced but progressively less intense (Fig. 1.14). This artifact may also be seen when the incident wave strikes smaller reflective objects such as the gas-fluid mixture in the small bowel. This results in a hyperechoic reflection distal to the structure with progressive attenuation of the sound wave (Fig. 1.15).

Reverberation artifact is often seen posterior to bowel (which contains air bubbles).

Correcting for Reverberation Artifact

Reverberation artifact may be overcome by changing the angle of insonation. When reverberation is caused by gas, compressing the abdominal wall with the probe may help to displace some of the gas.

Modes of Ultrasound

The most common modes of ultrasound used in clinical urological ultrasound are gray-scale (B-mode ultrasound) and Doppler ultrasound.

Gray-scale ultrasound

Gray-scale ultrasound images are produced when ultrasound waves are transmitted in a timed and sequential way (pulsed wave). The time of travel and degree of attenuation of the wave are reflected by the position on the monitor and the intensity by "brightness", respectively, of the corresponding pixel. Each sequential echo is displayed as a vertical line of pixels side-by-side and the entire image refreshed at 15–40 frames/s. This results in the illusion of continuous motion or "real-time" scanning. The intensity of the reflected sound waves may vary by a factor of 10^{12} or 120 dB [3]. Ultrasound units internally process and compress ultrasound data to allow it to be displayed on a monitor. Evaluation of gray-scale imaging requires the ability to recognize the normal patterns of echogenicity from anatomic structures. Variations from these expected patterns of echogenicity may indicate disorders of anatomy or may represent artifacts.

Doppler ultrasound

The Doppler ultrasound Mode depends on the physical principle of frequency shift which occurs when a sound waves strikes a moving object. The frequency of sound waves will be shifted or changed based on the direction and velocity of the moving object they strike as well as the angle of insonation. This phenomenon allows for the characterization of motion; most commonly the motion of blood through vessels. Detecting flow may also be useful for detecting the flow of urine from the ureteral orifices. In pelvic ultrasound for example demonstration of flow by Doppler can distinguish a dilated ureter from a pelvic blood vessel.

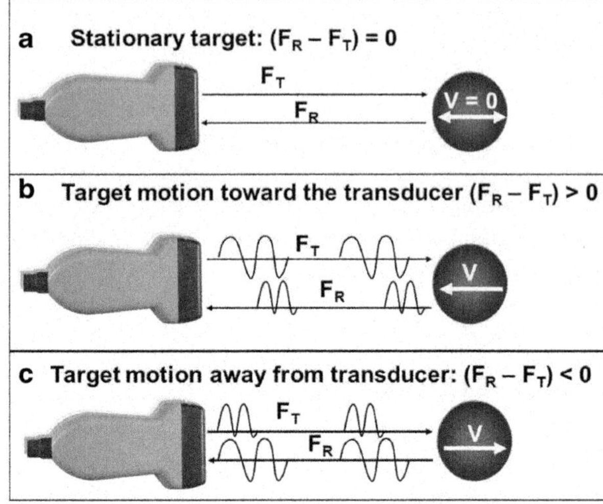

Fig. 1.16 Doppler effect. F_T is the transmitted frequency. When the F_T strikes a stationary object the returning frequency F_R is equal to the F_T (**a**). When the F_T strikes a moving object the F_R is "shifted" to a higher (**b**) or lower frequency (**c**)

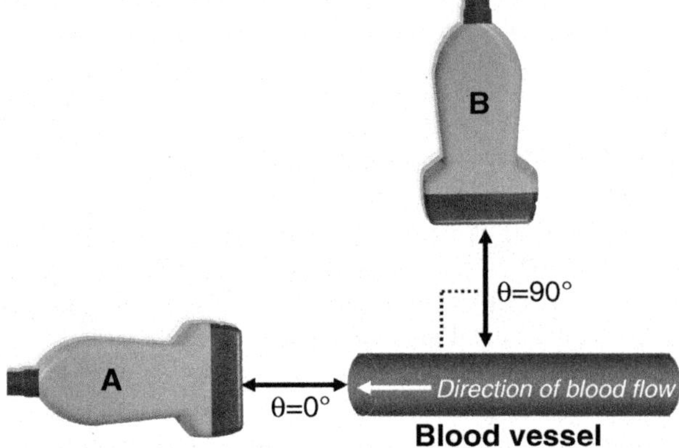

Fig. 1.17 Maximum frequency shifts are detected when the transducer axis is parallel to the direction of motion Angle θ = 0° (*A*). No frequency shift is detected when the transducer axis is perpendicular to the direction of motion Angle θ = 90° (*B*)

Doppler effect

The Doppler effect is a shift in the frequency of the transmitted sound wave based on the velocity and direction of the reflecting object that it strikes. If the reflecting object is stationary relative to the transducer then the returning frequency will be equal to the transmitted frequency. However, if the echo-generating object is traveling towards the transducer the returning frequency will be higher than the transmitted frequency. If the object generating the echo is traveling away from the transducer then the reflected frequency will be lower than the transmitted frequency. This is known as the frequency shift, or "Doppler shift" (Fig. 1.16).

The frequency shift of the transmitted wave is also dependent on the angle of the transducer relative to the object in motion. The maximum Doppler frequency shift occurs when the transducer is oriented directly on the axis of motion of the object

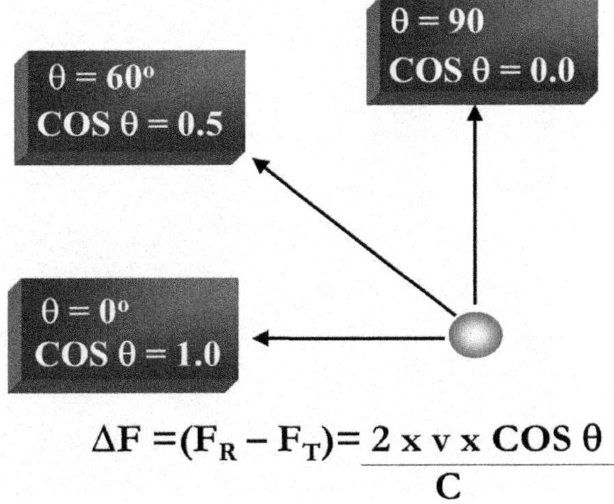

Fig. 1.18 Angle of insonation. The calculated velocity of an object using Doppler shift is dependent on the transducer angle (θ). If the transducer axis is perpendicular to the direction of flow (90°) then the cosign of θ is 0 (A). Based on this formula for Doppler shift (ΔF), the detected frequency change would be 0 (Adapted from *Radiographics*. 1991;11:109–119)

being insonated. That is, when the transducer is oriented parallel (angle θ=0°) to the direction of motion, the shift is maximal. Conversely, when the transducer face is oriented perpendicular to the direction of motion (angle θ=90°) there will be no shift in Doppler frequency detected regardless of the transmitted frequency (Fig. 1.17).

An accurate representation of velocity of flow depends on the angle (θ) between the transducer and the axis of motion of the object being insonated (Fig. 1.18). The angle should be less than or equal to 60° to minimize the error in calculation of the frequency shift.

Color Doppler

Color Doppler ultrasonography allows for an evaluation of the velocity and direction of an object in motion. A color map may be applied to the direction. The most common color map uses blue for motion away from the transducer and red for motion toward the transducer (Fig. 1.19).

The velocity of motion is designated by the intensity of the color. The greater the velocity of the motion, the brighter is the color displayed. Color Doppler may be used to characterize blood flow in the kidney, testis, penis and prostate. In pelvic imaging Color Doppler may be useful in the detection of "jets" of urine emerging from the ureteral orifices (Fig. 1.20).

An accurate representation of flow characteristics requires attention to transducer orientation relative to the object in motion. Therefore, in most clinical circumstances the angle between the transducer and the direction of motion should be less than or equal to 60° (Fig. 1.21).

When it is not possible to achieve an angle of 60° or less by manipulation of the transducer the beam may be "steered" electronically to help create the desired angle θ (Fig. 1.22).

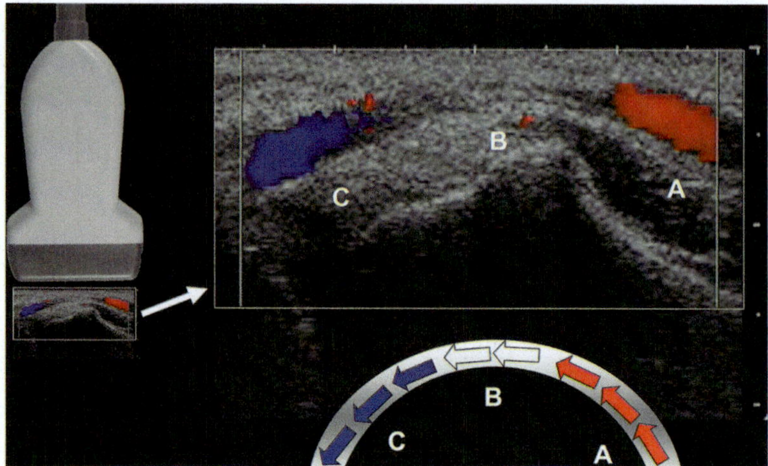

Fig. 1.19 In this image of the radial artery, blood is flowing through the curved vessel from *A* to *C*. (inset image designated by *arrow*) Flow towards the transducer (*A*) is depicted in *red*. Flow in the middle of the vessel (*B*) is perpendicular to the transducer axis and produces no Doppler shift thus, no color is assigned even though the velocity and intensity of flow are uniform through the vessel. Flow away from the transducer (*C*) is depicted in *blue*

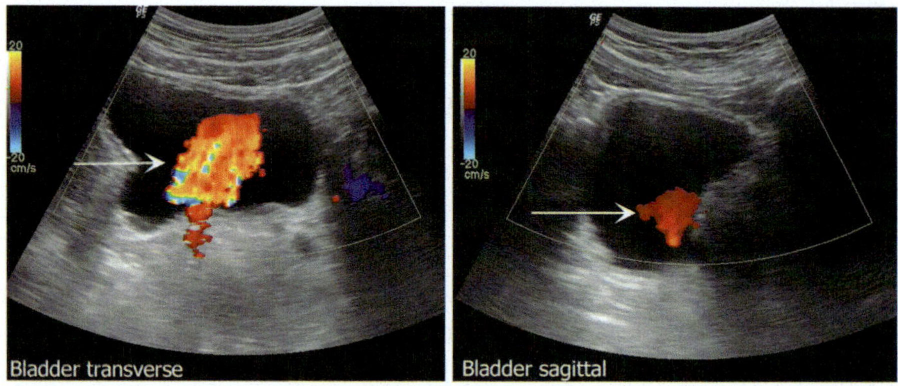

Fig. 1.20 Ureteral jets (*arrows*) appear *red* or *orange* in these color Doppler images since the urine is flowing towards the transducer

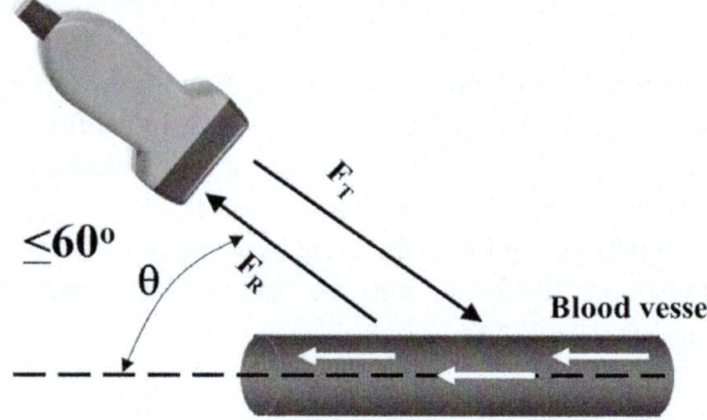

Fig. 1.21 The transducer angle should be ≤60° relative to the axis of fluid motion to allow a more accurate calculation of the velocity of flow

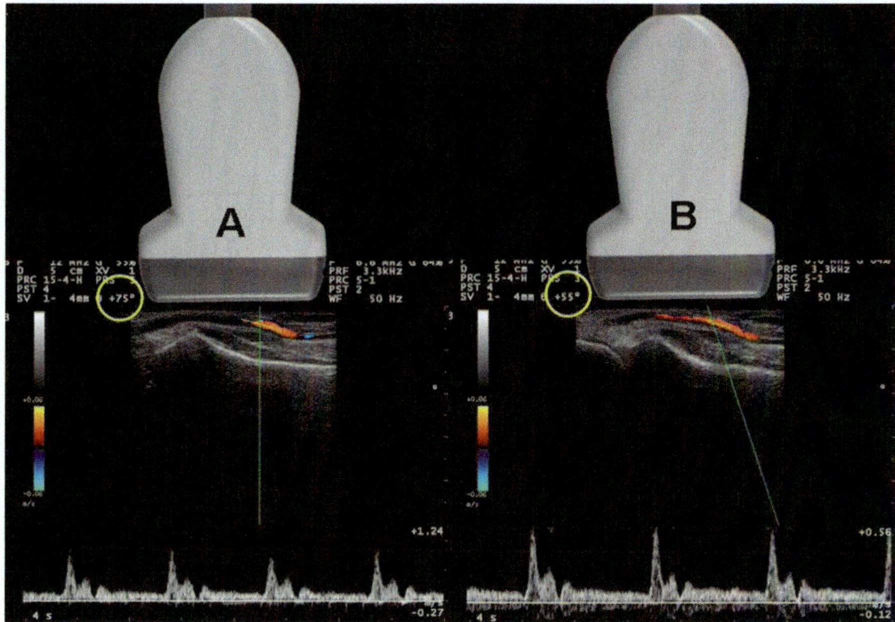

Fig. 1.22 Beam steering. In image (**a**) the angle of insonation is 75° (*yellow circle*) relative to the vessel which is unfavorable for accurate velocity calculations. This is because the axis of the transducer is perpendicular to the vessel. The beam angle is indicated by the *green line*. In image (**b**) the beam has been "steered" to produce an angle of 55° (*yellow circle*) without changing the physical position of the transducer. Note the beam angle (*green line*). The resultant velocity calculation is more accurate at 55°

Power Doppler

Power Doppler ultrasonography is a mode which assigns the amplitude of the waves associated with a given frequency shift to a color map. This does not permit evaluation of velocity or direction of flow but is less affected by back-scattered waves. Power Doppler is therefore less angle-dependent than color Doppler and is more sensitive for detecting flow [4].

When a sound wave strikes an object within the body, the sound wave is altered in a variety of ways including changes in frequency and changes in amplitude (Fig. 1.23).

While color Doppler assigns the changes in frequency to a color map, power Doppler assigns changes in integrated amplitude (or power) to a color map. It is possible to assign low level back scattered information to a color which is unobtrusive on the color map, thereby allowing increased gain without interference from this backscattered information (Fig. 1.24). Power Doppler may be more sensitive than color Doppler for the detection of diminished flow [4].

The integrated amplitude (power) of the Doppler signal is signified by the brightness of the color. Because the positive and negative frequency shifts are not assigned a unique corresponding color on the color map in standard power Doppler the direction and velocity of flow are not indicated. Power Doppler may be useful in the interrogation of tissues where there is relatively low blood flow (e.g. prostate, testes and ovaries).

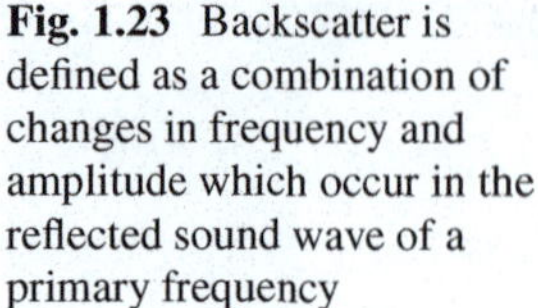

Fig. 1.23 Backscatter is defined as a combination of changes in frequency and amplitude which occur in the reflected sound wave of a primary frequency

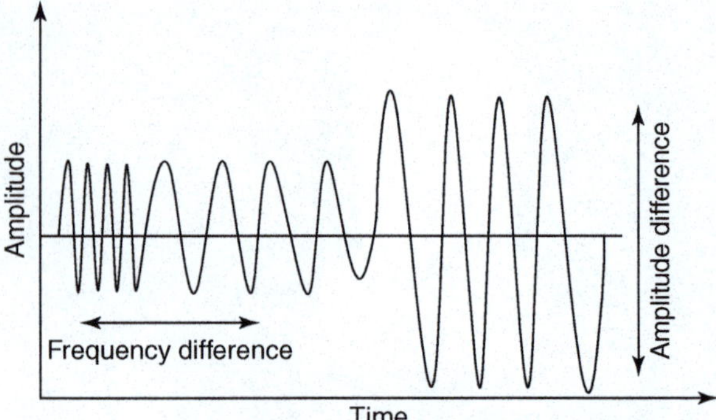

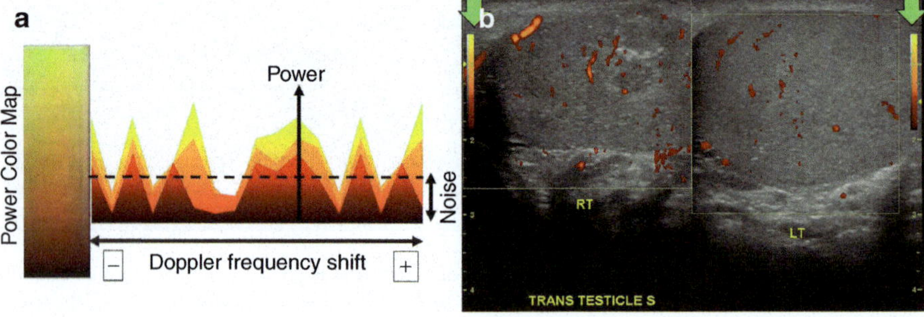

Fig. 1.24 (**a**) For power Doppler the intensity of color is related to changes in amplitude (power) rather than changes in frequency. (**b**) In this image of the testes, power Doppler blood flow is demonstrated. Note that the color maps depicted (*green arrows*) do not have a scale since a quantitative measurement of velocity is not displayed with standard power Doppler

Color Doppler with spectral display

Color Doppler with spectral display is a mode which allows the simultaneous display of a color Doppler image mapped onto the gray scale image and a representation of flow as a wave form within a discrete area of interrogation. This mode is commonly used to evaluate the pattern and velocity of blood flow in the kidney and testis (Fig. 1.25).

The spectral waveform provides information about peripheral vascular resistance in the tissues. The most commonly used index of these velocities is the resistive index (Fig. 1.26).

The resistive index may be helpful in characterizing a number of clinical conditions including renal artery stenosis and ureteral obstruction. Since the velocity is represented on a scaler axis, it is necessary to set appropriate scaler limits and adjust the pulse repetition frequency to prevent artifacts. Therefore, it is necessary to know the expected velocity within vessels pertinent to urologic practice (Table 1.2). The clinical use of resistive index is described in subsequent chapters.

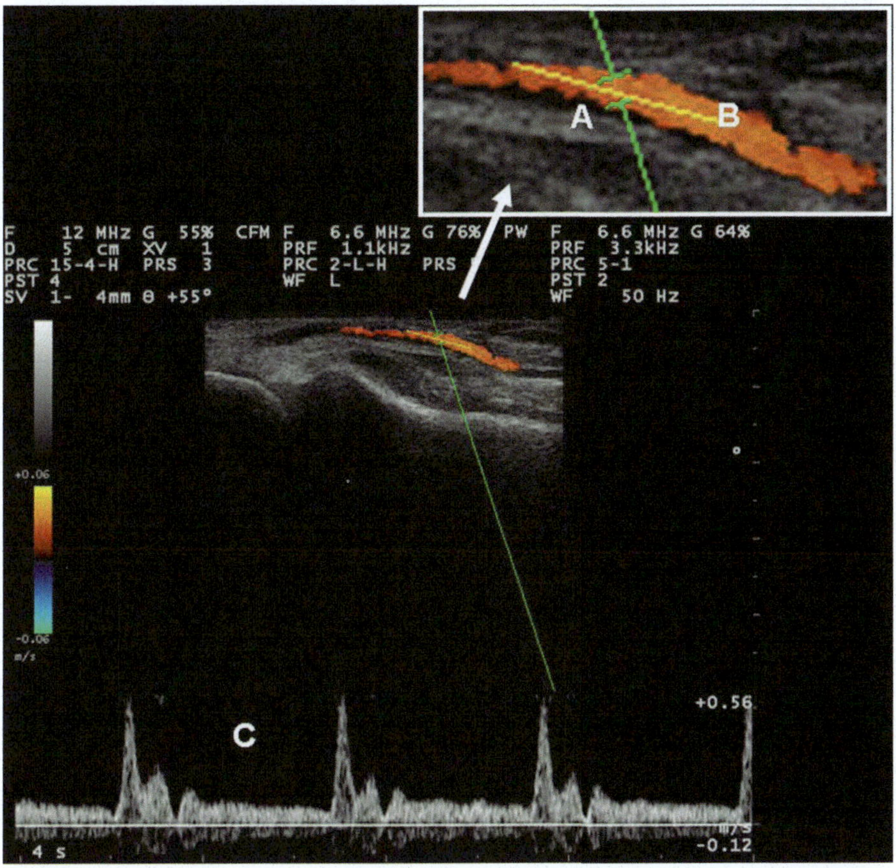

Fig. 1.25 In this example, (inset indicated by *arrow*) the radial artery is shown in real-time gray scale ultrasound with color Doppler overlay. The interrogation box or gate (*A*) is positioned over the vessel of interest. The gate should be positioned and sized to cover about 75 % of the lumen of the vessel. The angle of insonation is indicated by marking the orientation of the vessel with a cursor (*B*). The velocity of the flow within the vessel is depicted quantitatively in the spectral display (*C*)

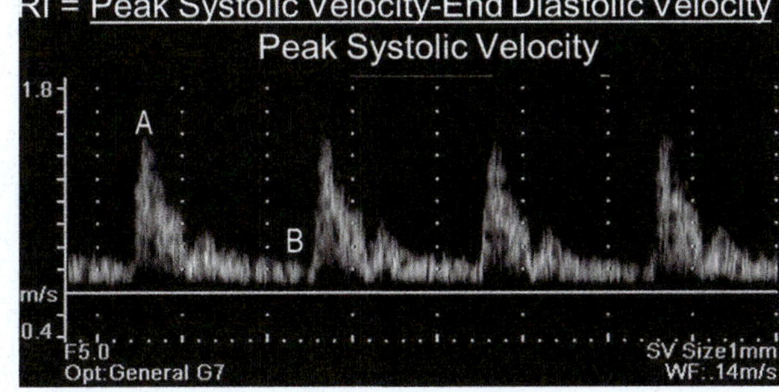

Fig. 1.26 The resistive index (*RI*) is the peak systolic velocity (*A*) minus the end-diastolic velocity (*B*) over the peak systolic velocity (*A*)

Table 1.2 Expected velocity in urologic vessels

Vessel	Velocity
Penile artery	>35 cm/s (after vasodilators) [5]
Renal artery	<100 cm/s [6]
Scrotal capsular artery	5–14 cm/s [7]

The measured velocity will depend on a variety of physiologic conditions and anatomic variants

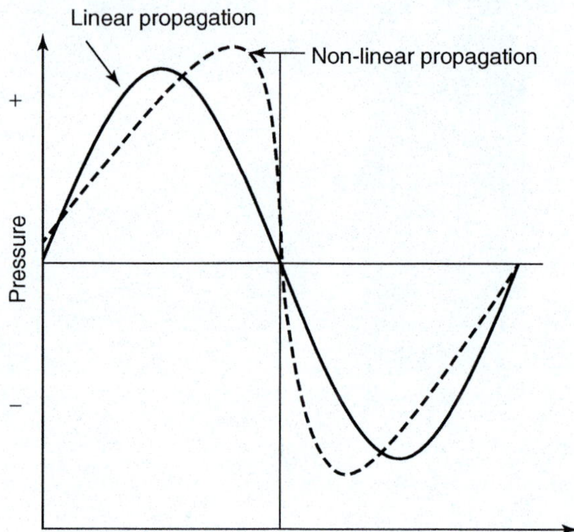

Fig. 1.27 Non-linear propagation of sound waves in tissue results in fewer but more energetic harmonics which may be selectively evaluated in the returning echo

Harmonic Scanning

Harmonic scanning makes use of aberrations related to the non-linear propagation of sound waves within tissue. These asymmetrically propagated waves generate fewer harmonics but those which are generated have greater amplitudes (Fig. 1.27).

Since these harmonics are less subject to scattering associated with the incident wave there is less noise associated with the signal. By selectively displaying the harmonic frequencies which are produced within the body and reflected to the transducer, it is possible to produce an image with less artifact. Harmonic imaging is often a useful tool in improving the image quality in obese patients.

Spatial compounding

Spatial compounding is a scanning mode whereby the direction of insonation is sequentially altered electronically to produce a composite image. This technique reduces the amount of artifact and noise producing a scan of enhanced clarity [8] (Fig. 1.28).

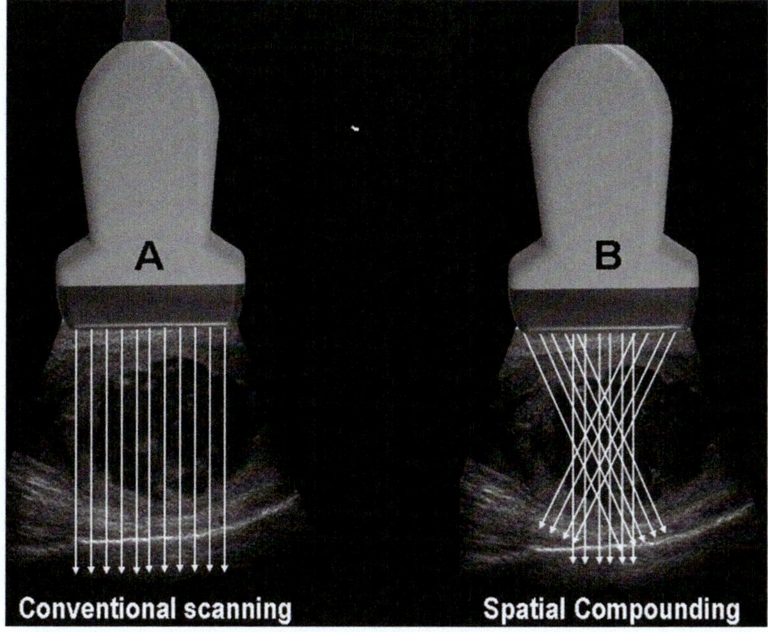

Fig. 1.28 Conventional scanning (**A**) constructs an image from echoes transmitted and received from a single angle. Spatial compounding (**B**) results in a composite image by combining data from multiple scanning angles produced by automated beam steering. The resulting image is more detailed with less artifact

Artifacts Associated with Doppler Ultrasound

Twinkle artifact

The twinkle artifact is produced when a sound wave encounters an interface which reflects and scatters the sound wave. Recent studies have shown that twinkle artifact is more likely to be produced by a reflective object with an irregular surface [9]. In the power and color Doppler mode this pattern of reflection gives the appearance of motion distal to that interface. The resulting Doppler signal appears as a trailing acoustic pattern of varying intensity and direction known as twinkle artifact. Although this artifact may be seen in a variety of clinical circumstances it is most often helpful clinically in evaluating hyperechoic objects in the kidney. Stones often demonstrate a twinkle artifact whereas arcuate vessels and other hyperechoic structures in the kidney usually do not. Calcifications of the renal artery and calcifications within tumors and cysts may also produce the twinkle artifact, though less consistently than stones [10]. Corpora amylacea in the prostate on transrectal ultrasound may produce the twinkle artifact (Fig. 1.29).

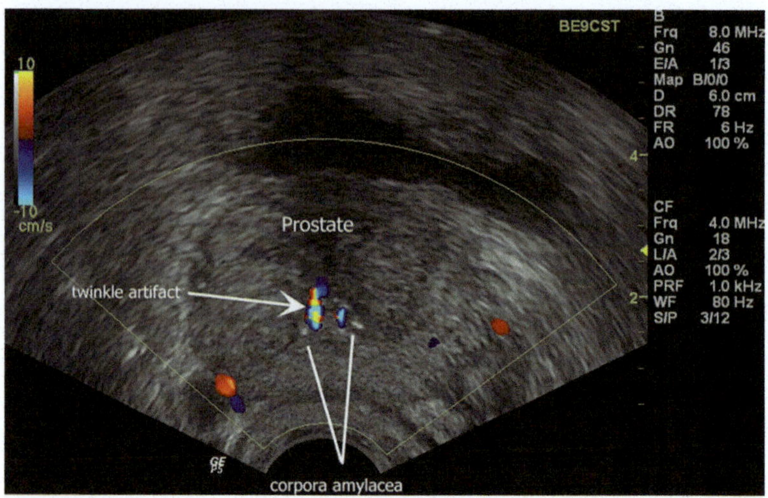

Fig. 1.29 Twinkle artifact. The effect produced by the interaction of sound waves at an interface with high impedance differences which produces an artifact suggesting turbulent motion (*arrow*). In this transverse transrectal ultrasound image of the prostate the twinkle artifact is produced by corpora amylacea (*thin arrows*)

Aliasing

Aliasing is an artifact which occurs when the ultrasound interrogation (determined by pulse repetition frequency) of an event occurs at a frequency which is insufficient to accurately represent the event. When interrogation occurs at infrequent intervals, only portions of the actual event are depicted. Aliasing occurs when the interrogation frequency is less than twice the shifted Doppler frequency (Fig. 1.30).

Normal laminar unidirectional blood flow is depicted as a single color on color Doppler. In this circumstance, spectral Doppler shows a complete waveform (Fig. 1.31). During color Doppler scanning, aliasing is most commonly seen as apparent turbulence and change in direction of blood flow within a vessel. During spectral Doppler scanning the aliasing phenomenon is seen as truncation of the systolic velocity peak with projection of the peak below the baseline (Fig. 1.32).

This artifact can be overcome by decreasing the frequency of the incident sound wave, increasing the angle of insonation (θ) or increasing the pulse repetition frequency (PRF).

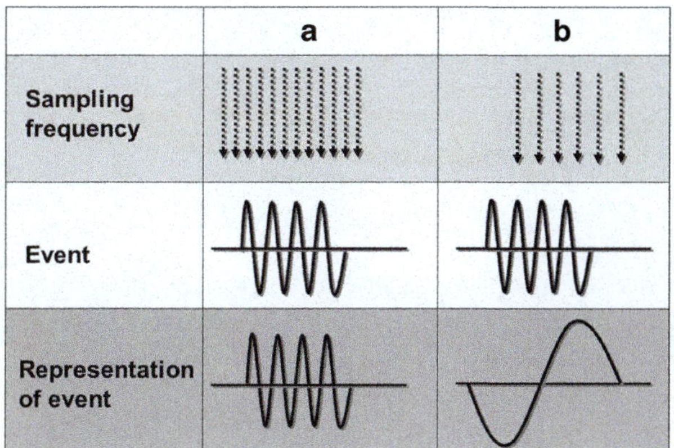

Fig. 1.30 Aliasing. In this illustration where a sine wave is the real-time event and the *vertical arrows* represent the frequency of interrogation we see that frequent interrogation produces an accurate representation of the event (**a**). An accurate depiction of an ultrasound event must meet the condition: $f_s \geq 2b$, where f_s is the sampling frequency and 2b is the highest frequency in the event. This is known as the Nyquist limit. (**b**) When the interrogation frequency is inadequate, the penetration of the event is inaccurate (Diagram adapted from *Diagnostic Ultrasound*, 3rd ed., Fig. 1–40, p. 33)

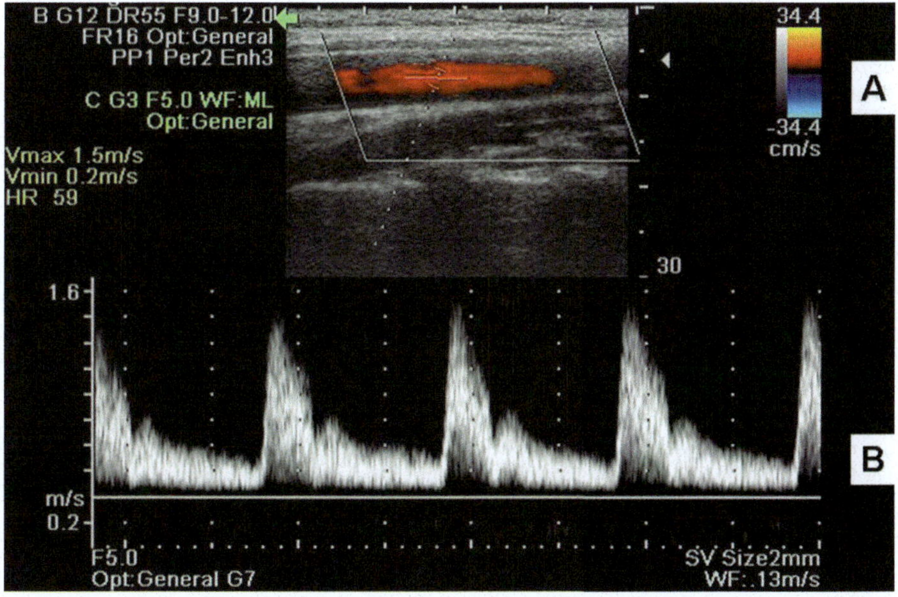

Fig. 1.31 Spectral Doppler. (**a**) Blood flow appears unidirectional on color mapping in this color Doppler image with spectral flow analysis. (**b**) The waveform is accurately depicted on spectral analysis

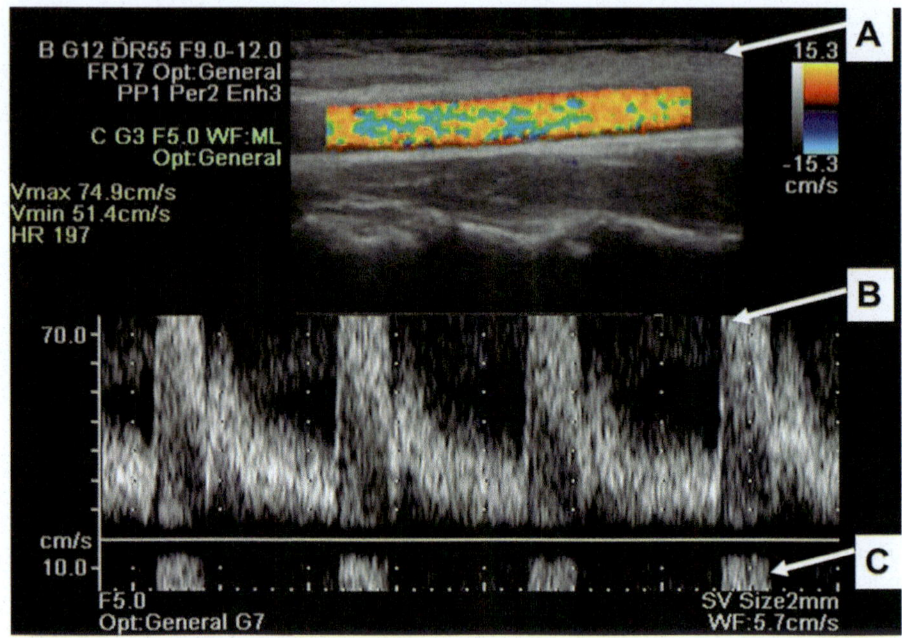

Fig. 1.32 In this color Doppler ultrasound with spectral flow, aliasing is demonstrated by apparent changes in velocity and direction on the color map assigned to the vessel in panel (**a**) indicated by *arrow*. Aliasing of the spectral waveform is seen as truncation of the peak systolic velocity in panel (**b**) as indicated by *arrow* with projection of the peak below the baseline in panel (**c**) as indicated by *arrow*

References

1. Mason WP. Piezoelectricity, its history and applications. J Acoust Soc Am. 1981;70(6): 1561–6.
2. Rumack CM, Wilson SR, Charboneau JW. Diagnostic ultrasound. 3rd ed. St. Louis: William. Mosby, Inc; 2005. p. 8.
3. Rumack CM, Wilson SR, Charboneau JW. Diagnostic ultrasound. 3rd ed. St. Louis: William. Mosby, Inc; 2005. p. 10.
4. Rubin JM, Bude RO, Carson PL, et al. Power Doppler US: a potentially useful alternative to mean frequency-based color Doppler US. Radiology. 1994;190:853–6.
5. Rifkin MD, Cochlin DL. Imaging of the scrotum & penis. Martin Dunitz Ltd; London, 2002. p. 276.
6. Zucchelli PC. Hypertension and atherosclerotic renal artery stenosis: diagnostic approach. J Am Soc Nephrol. 2002;13:S184–6.
7. Bluth EI, Benson CB, Ralls PW. Ultrasonography in vascular diseases: a practical approach to clinical problems. Thieme Medical Publishers; New York, 2008. p. 87.
8. Merritt CR. Technology update. Radiol Clin North Am. 2001;39:385–97.
9. Sharma G, Sharma A. Clinical implications and applications of the twinkling sign in ureteral calculus: a preliminary study. J Urol. 2013;189:2132–5.
10. Kim HC, Yang DM, Wook J, Jung Kyu R, Hyeong Cheol S. Color Doppler twinkling artifacts in various conditions during abdominal and pelvic sonography. J Ultrasound Med. 2010; 29:621–32.

Chapter 2
Machine Settings and Technique of Image Optimization

Pat F. Fulgham

Ultrasound machine settings may be adjusted in order to obtain a good quality image. These settings include but are not limited to gain, time-gain compensation, frequency, focal zones, depth/size, field of view and cine function. A good quality ultrasound image will have sufficient and uniform brightness. It will be sharp and the focal zones will be set at the area of interest. The area of interest will be of adequate size and will be oriented properly and labeled for documentation purposes (Fig. 2.1).

Transducer Selection

The first step in performing ultrasound is to select the transducer with the optimal shape. A linear-array transducer produces a rectangular image and is generally used for scrotal ultrasound (Fig. 2.2). A curved-array transducer produces an image which is trapezoidal in shape and is generally used for abdominal and pelvic ultrasound (Fig. 2.2). The curved nature of the probe allows gentle pressure on the patient's abdomen or flank resulting in contact of the entire transducer face with the skin. Endocavitary probes (transvaginal and transrectal probes) are curved array probes with trapezoidal image displays.

Transducers are usually multifrequency, meaning the frequency can be switched electronically over a range of frequencies (e.g. 3.5–5.0 mHz for transabdominal pelvic ultrasound). It is important to select the highest frequency which has adequate depth of penetration for the anatomic area of interest. The higher the frequency the greater the axial resolution and the better the anatomic representation of the image. However, the higher the frequency the lower the depth of penetration (Fig. 2.3).

P.F. Fulgham, MD, DABU, FACS
Department of Urology, Texas Health Presbyterian Hospital of Dallas,
8210 Walnut Hill Suite 014, Dallas, TX 75231, USA
e-mail: pfulgham@airmail.net

L. Chan et al. (eds.), *Pelvic Floor Ultrasound: Principles, Applications and Case Studies*, DOI 10.1007/978-3-319-04310-4_2

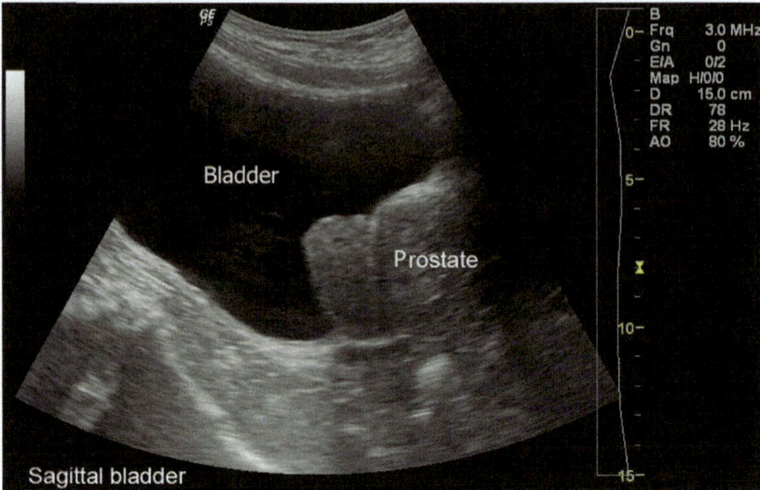

Fig. 2.1 This image displays the characteristics of a good quality image by virtue of technical settings of user-controlled variables as well as proper labeling

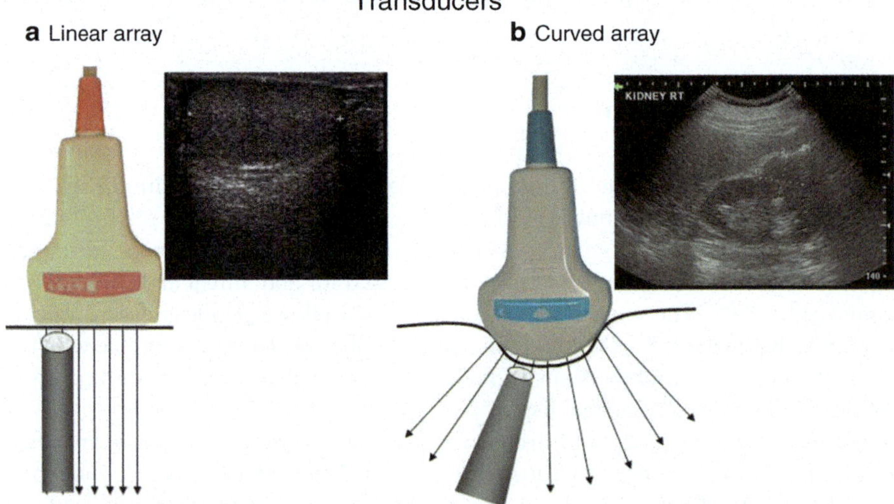

Fig. 2.2 (**a**) The linear array transducer produces a rectangular image field. (**b**) The curved array transducer produces a trapezoidal or pie-shaped image. The shape of the transducer affects the divergence of the wave as the wave propagates in the body

Scanning Environment

To produce the best quality image the sonographer should arrange the scanning environment so that access to the patient and equipment are optimized (Fig. 2.4). The table should be positioned at a height which allows the sonographer to stand or

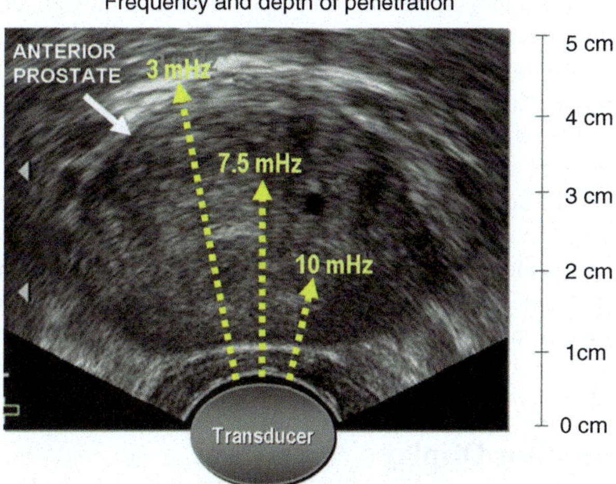

Fig. 2.3 The selection of a transducer with the frequency of 7.5 mHz reflects the trade off between depth of penetration and good axial resolution. In this axial image of a large prostate, a lower scanning frequency may be needed to adequately visualize the anterior prostate

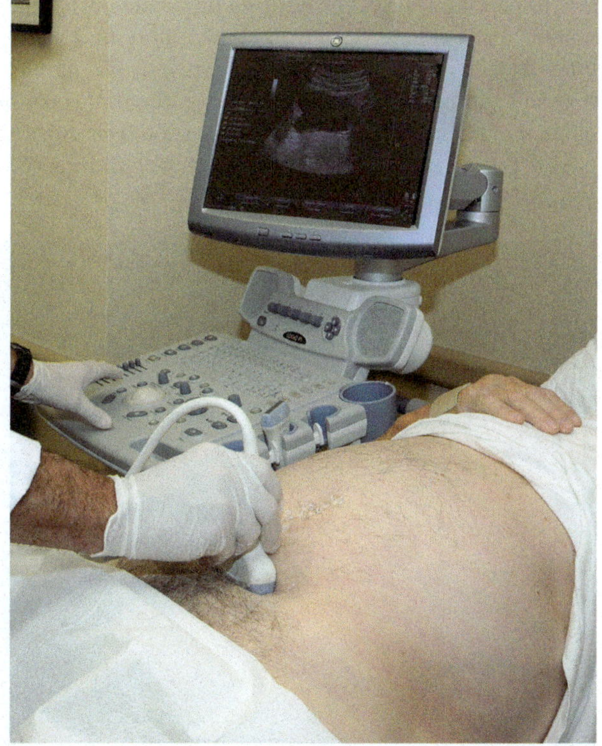

Fig. 2.4 The configuration of the equipment and proximity to the patient are critical in maximizing comfort, efficiency, and accuracy during scanning and documentation

sit in a comfortable position so that the sonographer is able to stabilize the transducer against the patient's body. This minimizes unwanted movement of the transducer and allows the sonographer to maintain the orientation and position of the transducer while adjusting machine features.

The sonographer should be positioned so they are able to comfortably reach the physical console or touch screen in order to adjust the machine settings. Many ultrasound units provide the ability to freeze and unfreeze the transducer via a button on the transducer itself or by a footswitch. In either case the sonographer must be able to scan the patient with one hand while manipulating the console and documenting with the other hand.

The sonographer must have a clear direct view of the monitor. The angle of the monitor should be adjusted for viewing by the sonographer. The brightness settings on the monitor need to be adjusted for the conditions under which the scan is being performed. In general, dimming the room lights improves the ability to evaluate the image on the monitor.

Monitor Display

It is important when performing an ultrasound examination to understand the information that is being displayed on the monitor. Patient demographic information, type of exam and facility should be entered. The monitor will usually display information regarding which probe is active, the frequency of the probe, and the magnification of the image (Fig. 2.5). Information regarding overall gain and other settings is available on the monitor. Typically there will be a TGC (time-gain compensation)

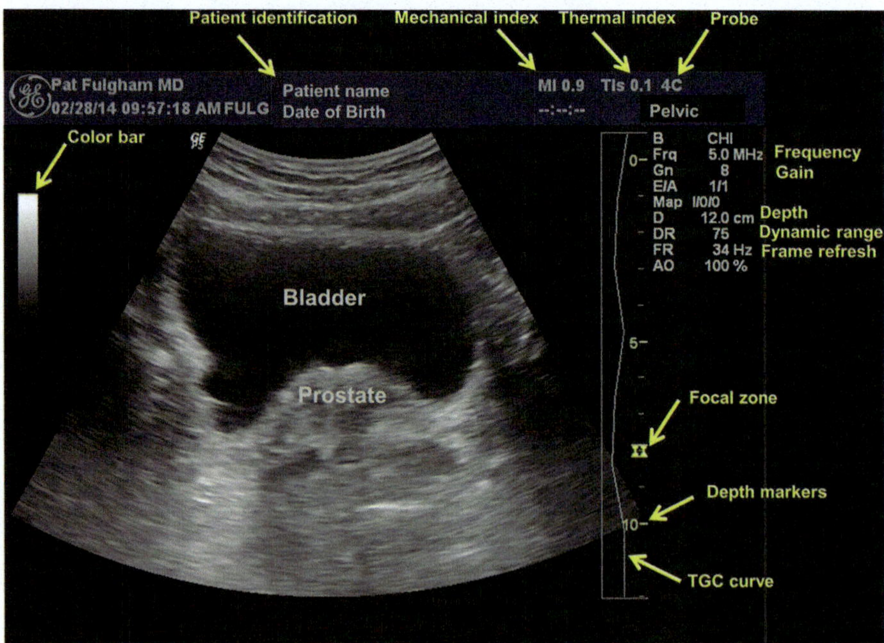

Fig. 2.5 Machine settings and icons displayed on the monitor help with adjusting machine settings to optimize image quality

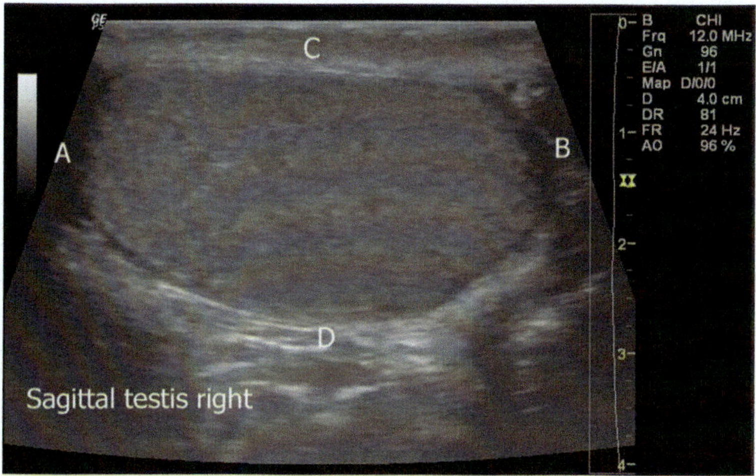

Fig. 2.6 In this sagittal image of the right testis, the superior pole of the testis (*A*) is to the *left*, the inferior pole of the testis (*B*) is to the *right*. The anterior aspect of the testis (*C*) is at the *top* of the image and the posterior aspect (*D*) at the *bottom*. Without the label (Sagittal testis *right*) there would be no way to distinguish the right from the left testis

curve displayed on one side of the image as well as color bar which demonstrates the range of pixel brightness or hues available. In addition, there will be gradient markings on one side so that depth of field can be appreciated.

Orientation

By convention, when scanning organs in the sagittal view, the upper pole of the organ (e.g. kidney or testis) is to the left of the screen and the lower pole is to the right of the screen (Fig. 2.6).

In transverse scanning the right side of an anatomic structure is displayed on the left side of the image just as it would be when evaluating a conventional radiograph. These conventions should always be followed when documenting an ultrasound examination; however, it may be useful to also demonstrate the orientation of the probe using graphics or icons. When paired structures such as the kidneys or testes are imaged it is particularly important to designate the organ as right or left.

User-Controlled Variables

One of the most commonly required adjustments during ultrasound scanning is an adjustment to the overall **gain**. The gain is a control which determines the degree to which the electrical signal produced by a returning sound wave when it strikes the transducer will be amplified for display. This needs to be differentiated from

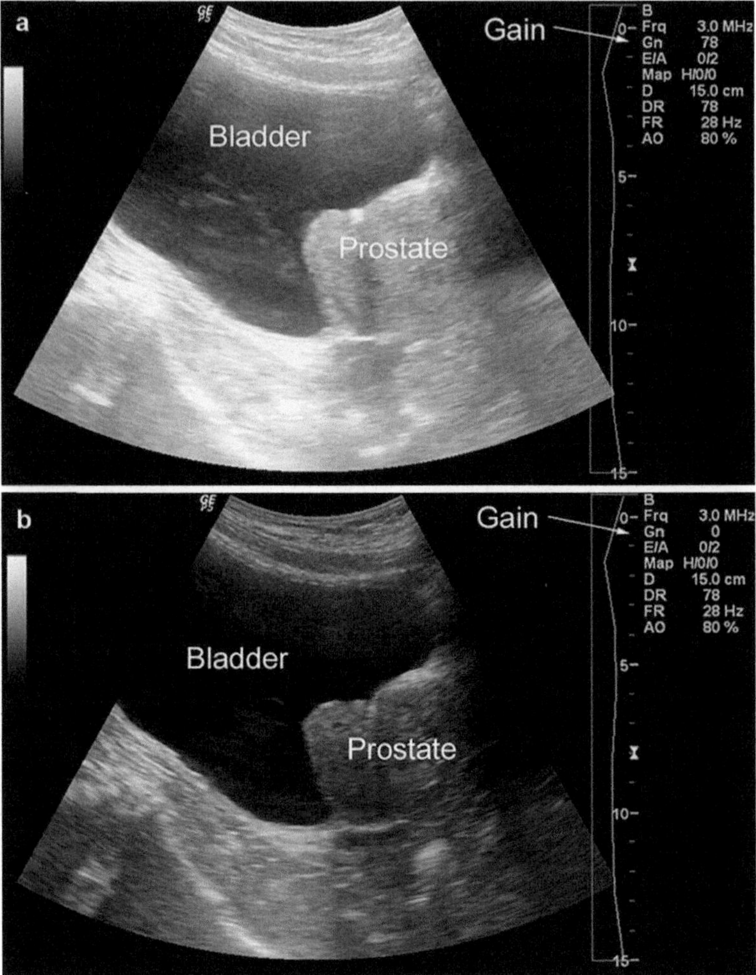

Fig. 2.7 In this sagittal view of the bladder and prostate, (**a**) demonstrates a gain setting which produces bright echoes throughout the image, accentuating slice thickness artifact seen in the anterior bladder and obscuring the detail of the tissues posterior to the bladder because of increased through-transmission. (**b**) Demonstrates an overall gain setting which results in good contrast, less artifact and better overall tissue detail

acoustic output which is defined as the power or amplitude of the afferent wave which is generated by the transducer.

Both gain and acoustic power can be controlled by the operator; however, acoustic output is limited by the manufacturer in compliance with industry safety standards [1]. In general, when the gain is increased the resulting image is brighter. When there is excessive overall gain the image often appears bright and washed out. When there is insufficient overall gain the image is often dark and it is difficult to distinguish between adjacent structures (Fig. 2.7).

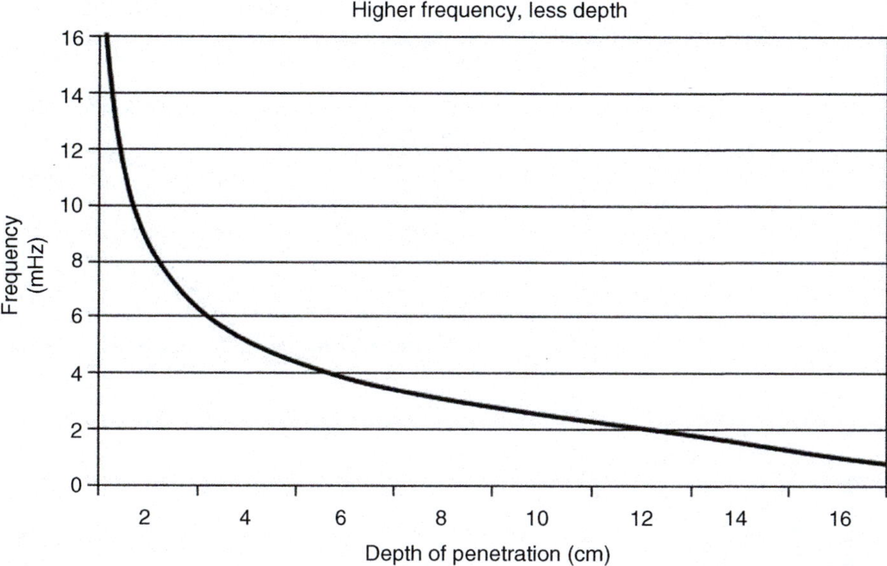

Fig. 2.10 The relative relationship between frequency and depth of penetration. Notice that to image a kidney 12 cm beneath the skin, a frequency of 2–4 mHz would be required to achieve an adequate depth of penetration

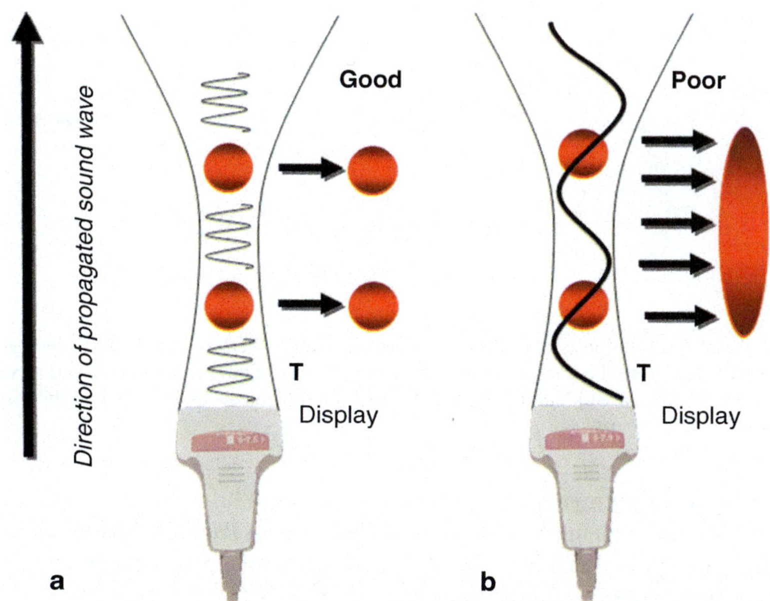

Fig. 2.11 (**a**) The shorter pulse length associated with this higher frequency wave is able to fit between the two objects in the axial plane providing good axial resolution. (**b**) The longer pulse length is unable to fit between the objects, thus depicting the two distinct objects as a single "blurred" echogenic focus

Fig.2.12 An example of calculating the axial resolution for a 5 mHz probe

Axial resolution for a 5 mHz Probe

1 pulse = 3λ

$v=f\lambda$

For normal tissue velocity of 1540 m/sec and a frequency of 5 mHz

$\lambda=v/f$

λ=1,540 m/s / 5mHz

λ=0.34 mm

3λ=1.02 mm

∴ 1 pulse = 1.02 mm

Therefore, axial resolution at 5 mHz ≥ 1.02 mm

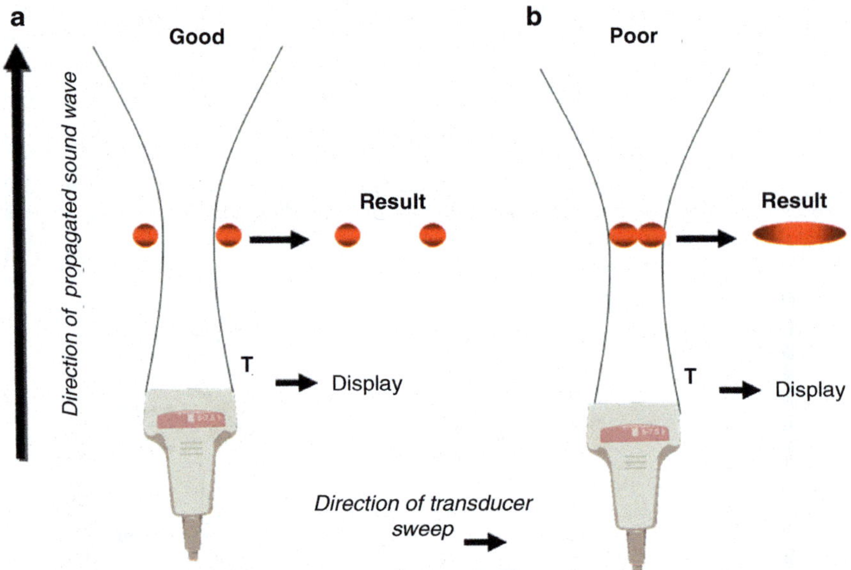

Fig.2.13 Lateral resolution is optimized when beam width is narrow enough to fit between two objects equidistant from the transducer. In (**a**) the objects would be correctly displayed as separate objects. In (**b**) the beam width is too thick to fit between the objects and they would be displayed as a single "blurred" focus

Focal zone adjustments are made in an attempt to bring the narrowest portion of the ultrasound beam into the location where maximal lateral resolution is desired. Lateral resolution is defined as the ability to discriminate as separate, two points which are equidistance from the transducer (Fig. 2.13).

Lateral resolution is a function of the width of the sound wave beam. The more focused the beam the better the lateral resolution; that is, even closely spaced objects can be differentiated. Most transducers have a focal point producing the best lateral resolution and a focal range producing adequate lateral resolution (Fig. 2.14).

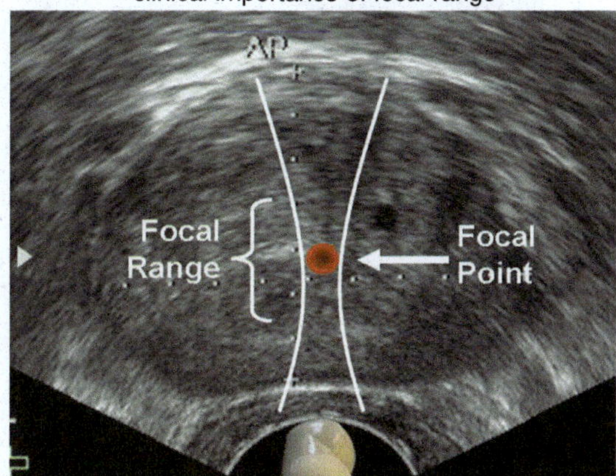

Fig. 2.14 The shape of the ultrasound beam determines its lateral resolution. The narrowest portions of the beam is its focal point or focal zone. The location of the narrowest point of the beam can be adjusted by manually setting foci

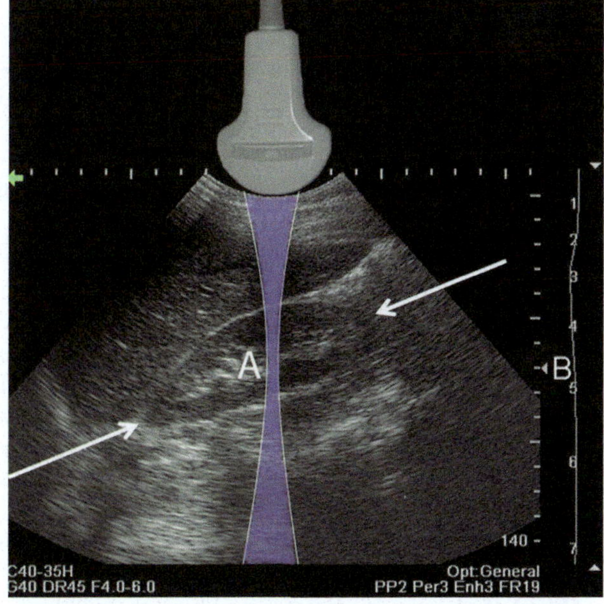

Fig. 2.15 The shape of the ultrasound beam is simulated in this drawing (*purple*). The focal zone (*A*) is located to produce the best lateral resolution of the medial renal cortex (*white arrows*). The location of the focal zone is designated by the *arrowhead* (*B*). The location of the focal zone can be adjusted by the operator

The location of the narrowest portion of the ultrasound beam can be set by adjusting the focal zone. However, the thickness of the beam (known as the elevation or Azimuth) is determined by the characteristics of the transducer crystals and design. In general, the focal zone should be placed at or just distal to the area that is of maximum clinical interest (Fig. 2.15).

It is possible to set multiple focal zones; however, this requires the software to sequentially interpret returning sound waves from specific locations of the scanning field (Fig. 2.16).

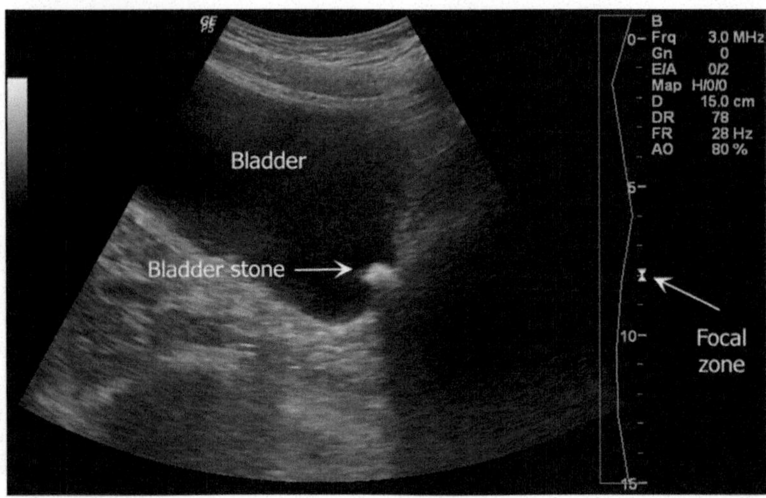

Fig. 2.16 In this sagittal view of the bladder the focal zone is set at the level of the bladder stone

Multiple focal zones result in a slower frame refresh rate and may result in a display motion that is discontinuous. In most urologic scanning applications a slower refresh rate is not a significant liability. Multiple focal zones are most useful in urologic scanning when fine anatomic detail throughout a solid structure is desirable (notably, in testicular scanning). When it is desirable to produce and interpret a twinkle artifact during Doppler scanning it is useful to place the focus just at or distal to the object producing the twinkle artifact.

Depth/size function allows the user to select that portion of the scanned field which will be displayed on the monitor. By adjusting the depth of field it is possible to allow the structure of interest to occupy the appropriate proportion of the visual field. By limiting the area of the scanned field from which returning echo signals will need to be interpreted and displayed the amount of work performed interpreting that returning information will be diminished and frame refresh rates will be improved. The depth/size function has no effect on the axial resolution of the image. Appropriate depth of field adjustments can improve the ability to visually discriminate certain structures during urologic scanning and improves the overall performance of the equipment (Fig. 2.17).

Field of view is an adjustment to limit the width of an image so that only a portion of the available ultrasound information is interpreted. As with changes in depth of field narrowing the field of view will reduce the amount of work necessary to interpret the returning echo data and improve frame refresh rate. It also limits the visual distraction of tissues which are irrelevant to a specific exam (Fig. 2.18).

The **cine function** of most machines provides an opportunity to save a sequence of frames from the most recent scanning session and allows these frames to be played back one by one. This is a very useful feature when scanning organs such as

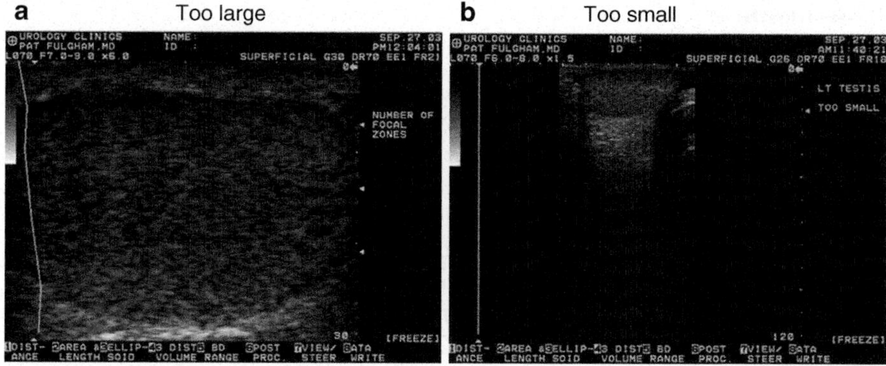

Fig. 2.17 (**a**) Depth of field has been set so that the testis fills the available display space but produces a grainy image. (**b**) Depth of field has been increased so that the testis occupies a very small portion of the available display. Tissue posterior to the testis which is not relevant, occupies a large percentage of the display

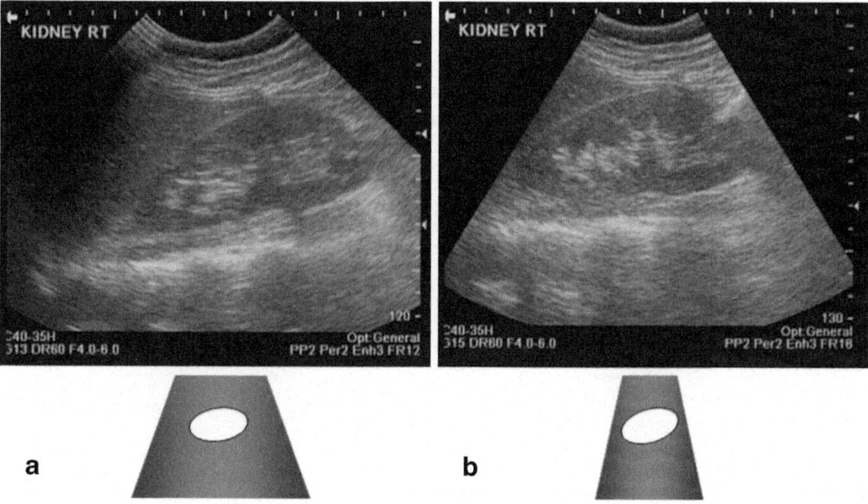

Fig. 2.18 The full ultrasound field is displayed in (**a**). Limiting the field of view to the kidney (**b**) decreases the time necessary to interpret returning echo information and improves the frame refresh rate

the kidney which may be affected by respiratory motion. When a subtle finding is identified the machine can be placed in the freeze mode and then the sequential images captured in the cine memory can be scanned backwards until the most appropriate image for measurement and documentation is identified. The cine function is invaluable in clinical office urology because it significantly decreases the time necessary to perform and document a complete examination.

Conclusion

Ultrasound is ultimately an exercise in image recognition. Clinicians tend to see what they know and that with which they are familiar. Great care must be taken to ensure optimal image quality so that the unexpected and unfamiliar may also be recognized and correctly diagnosed. While ultrasound equipment has preset applications which allow scanning of most patients without the need to make individual adjustments, there are many clinical circumstances in which the ability to make individual adjustments is invaluable for making a clinical diagnosis or clarifying an artifact. Knowledge of the physical properties of ultrasound and the judicious use of basic instrumental controls such as TGC, Depth, Gain and Focus will allow the clinician to maximize the diagnostic capability of this modality of imaging in evaluating pelvic floor disorders.

Reference

1. Guidance for industry and FDA staff information for manufacturers seeking marketing clearance of diagnostic ultrasound systems and transducers. Document issued on: 9 Sept 2008. http://www.fda.gov/downloads/MedicalDevices/DeviceRegulationandGuidance/GuidanceDocuments/UCM070911.pdf.

Chapter 3
Essentials for Setting Up Practice in Clinician Performed Ultrasound

Lewis Chan

Pelvic floor ultrasound is best performed by a clinician with detailed knowledge of the pathophysiology of pelvic floor function and dysfunction. Ultrasound imaging may be considered an extension of clinical examination or part of a functional assessment of voiding and pelvic floor dysfunction.

Nonetheless, as most clinicians (gynaecologists, urologists, colorectal surgeons physiotherapists) may not be performing diagnostic ultrasound imaging on a daily basis the choice of equipment and setup needs careful consideration. Potential environments in which a clinician may perform ultrasound include the office, hospital wards, clinics and formal radiology imaging facilities in a hospital or private setting.

Choosing Ultrasound Equipment

Selection of ultrasound equipment greatly depends on the needs of the user or users. In general, any ultrasound machine with B mode, grayscale scan capacity will be suitable for 2D pelvic floor ultrasound. The availability of color doppler function may be useful to look for flow in pelvic vessels and identify ureteric jets. 'Higher end' function such as 3D/4D function and volume analysis are more practical in larger clinical units where clinicians perform different types of scans. This may also be desirable if the clinicians' practice involves patients with complex voiding dysfunction, pelvic organ prolapse and mesh repairs. These machines are generally cart based but there are now portable ultrasound units with 3D functionality becoming increasingly available and affordable.

L. Chan, MBBS(Hons), FRACS, DDU
Department of Urology, Concord Repatriation General Hospital, Sydney, NSW, Australia
e-mail: lewis.chan@sswahs.nsw.gov.au

L. Chan et al. (eds.), *Pelvic Floor Ultrasound: Principles, Applications and Case Studies*, DOI 10.1007/978-3-319-04310-4_3

Portable Units Versus Trolley/Cart Based Systems

Portable ultrasound machines are advantageous if the clinician delivers care in different practice locations and are especially suitable for bedside ultrasound.

Transducer Selection

The appropriate number and types of transducers depend on the type of pelvic scanning in the clinician's practice. Most can start with a standard general purpose curved array (for example, a 2–5 MHz transducer for transabdominal and transperineal imaging) and an intracavity transducer for prostate and pelvic organ imaging. An endoanal transducer is important if anorectal sphincteric function assessment is planned.

Upgrade and software options are useful especially in larger units with higher end ultrasound machines where different types of ultrasound scans are performed.

Image recording options include thermal prints, digital output such as CD/DVD/USB recording, or a Picture Archiving and Communication System (PACS).

Equipment Setup, Maintainence and Protection

The most fragile part of the ultrasound unit is the transducer and this must be protected from drop damage (Fig. 3.1). It is also important to protect the electronics of the transducer coupling (Fig. 3.2) especially in the disinfection/sterilization of endocavity probes. No matter how simple the ultrasound equipment is, it is in the clinician's interest to be fully orientated to the features of the machine and be involved in creating the pre-set functions (see Chap. 2) to ensuring that the best possible images can be obtained during scanning.

Setting Up the Ultrasound Room

The physical environment in which pelvic floor ultrasound is performed can have significant impact on a patient's or sonographer's comfort and indirectly affect the quality of images and interpretation of the scan findings. This is especially because pelvic floor imaging is often performed as part of functional/dynamic assessment of pelvic floor dysfunction.

Both the examination table and the sonographer's chair should ideally be height adjustable. The physical configuration of the scanning room should ensure that the clinician has ready access to the ultrasound machine, examination table, gel, towels and lighting controls (Figs. 3.3 and 3.4). Space for a support person (for the patient) or chaperone is also important especially when performing intracavity imaging.

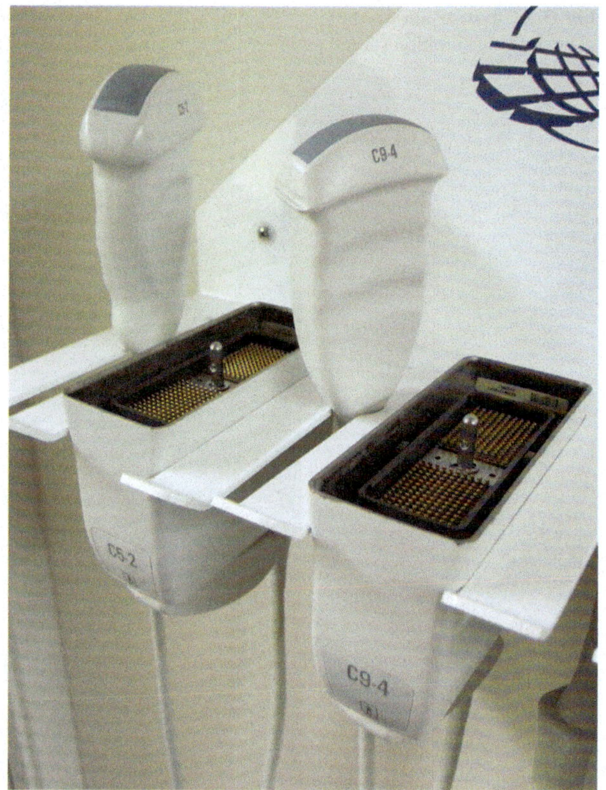

Fig. 3.1 The transducer is the most fragile part of the ultrasound unit and should be protected from drop damage during storage and scanning

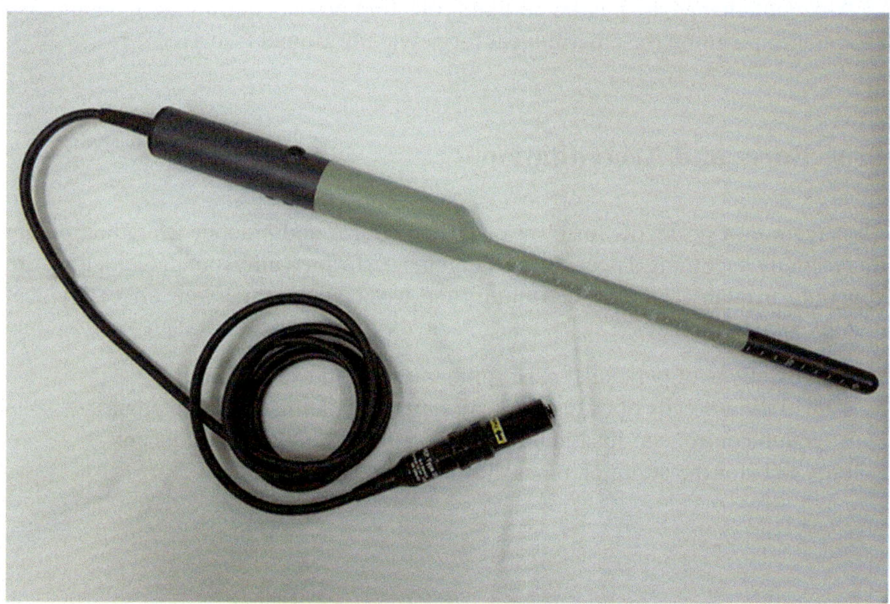

Fig. 3.2 During sterilization of intracavity transducers the transducer coupling should be protected

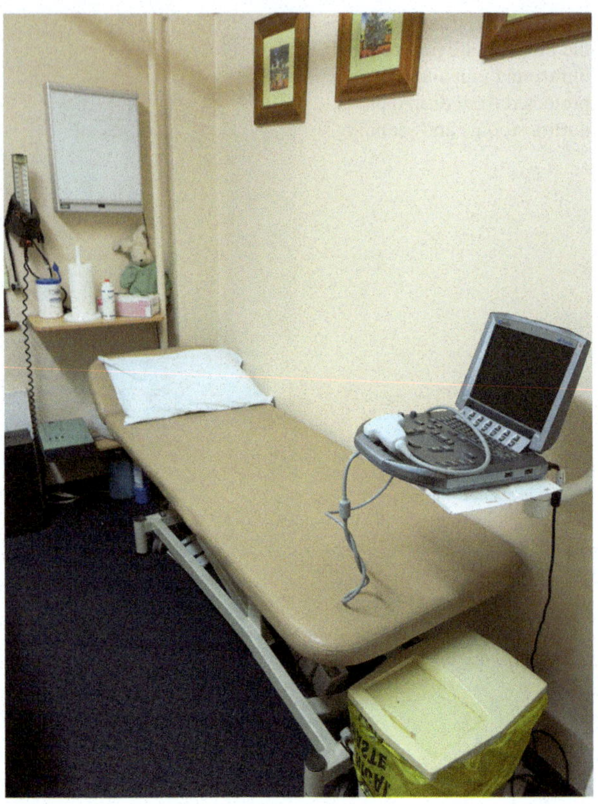

Fig. 3.3 Bedside ultrasound setup in a consultation room

A patient change area and a curtain protecting privacy during the scan are also essential in planning the environment for pelvic ultrasound (see Tips 3.1)

Procedures and Accreditation

The creation of protocols for ultrasound procedures and practice accreditation are increasingly becoming a necessity in clinician performed ultrasound. Guidelines are generally available via national ultrasound associations (see web links). Typical documentation includes:

- Qualifications of personnel performing ultrasound examinations
- Registration/details of ultrasound equipment, updating and maintenance
- Infection control, sterilisation/disinfection procedures for transducers
- Protocols for the common types of scans performed

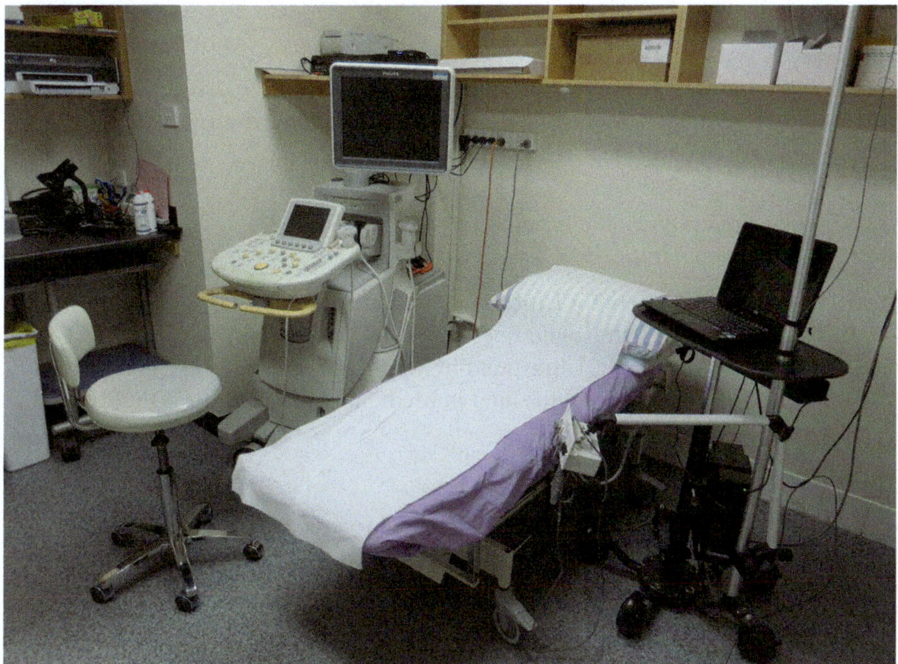

Fig. 3.4 Dedicated ultrasound room setup for pelvic floor imaging and ultrasound urodynamics

- Reporting format
- Referral format (if the clinician performs ultrasound scans for external referrers)
- Recording of images
- Availability of chaperones

Tips 3.1 Checklist for Setting Up the Ultrasound Room (Figs. 3.3 and 3.4)

Space and location

Bedside scanning arrangement

Easily accessible lighting and switches

Adjustable height examination couch

Comfortable, height adjustable chair for sonographer

Availability of toilet, change area and curtains

Appendix

A. ASUM statement on Disinfection of Transducers
   www.asum.com.au/newsite/files/documents/policies/PS/B2_policy.pdf
B. AIUM/AUA Practice Guidelines for Ultrasound Examination in the Practice of Urology
   www.aium.org/resources/guidelines/urology.pdf
C. Links to national ultrasound associations

   1. Australasian Society for Ultrasound in Medicine (ASUM) www.asum.com.au
   2. British Medical Ultrasound Society (BMUS) www.bmus.org
   3. American Institute of Ultrasound in Medicine (AIUM) www.aium.org
   4. World Federation for Ultrasound in Medicine and Biology (WFUMB) www.wfumb.org

Chapter 4
Ultrasound Imaging in Assessment of the Male Patient with Voiding Dysfunction

Lewis Chan, Tom Jarvis, Stuart Baptist, and Vincent Tse

Ultrasound imaging is often performed in the assessment of the male patient with lower urinary symptoms (LUTS) and voiding dysfunction. The male pelvis can be imaged by transabdominal, transperineal and transrectal approaches (Fig. 4.1). Urologists have a long history of performing transrectal ultrasound in the diagnosis and treatment of prostate cancer and this aspect of imaging is beyond the scope of this book. This chapter will focus on the application of transabdominal and transperineal ultrasound in the assessment of voiding dysfunction in the male patient.

Transabdominal Ultrasound

Transabdominal ultrasound of the pelvis can assist in the evaluation of bladder outlet obstruction, measurement of bladder volume, post-void residual, prostate volume, ureteric jets (Fig. 1.20) and other bladder pathology such as tumours or stones.

Electronic supplementary material The online version of this chapter (doi: 10.1007/978-3-319-04310-4_4) contains supplementary material, which is available to authorized users.

L. Chan, MBBS(Hons), FRACS, DDU (✉) • V. Tse, MBBS, MS, FRACS
Department of Urology, Concord Repatriation General Hospital, Sydney, NSW Australia
e-mail: lewis.chan@sswahs.nsw.gov.au; vincent.tse@sydney.edu.au

T. Jarvis, BSc(Med), MBBS(Hons), FRACS(Uro)
Department of Urology, Prince of Wales Hospital,
Barker Street, Randwick, NSW 2031, Australia
e-mail: tomjarvis@ozdoctors.com

S. Baptist, BSc (Hons)Physio, RPT, APAM, CFA
Sydney Sports and Orthopaedic Physiotherapy Group,
Level 1, 139 Macquarie Street, Sydney, NSW 2000, Australia
e-mail: stuartbaptist@ssop.com.au

L. Chan et al. (eds.), *Pelvic Floor Ultrasound: Principles, Applications and Case Studies*, DOI 10.1007/978-3-319-04310-4_4

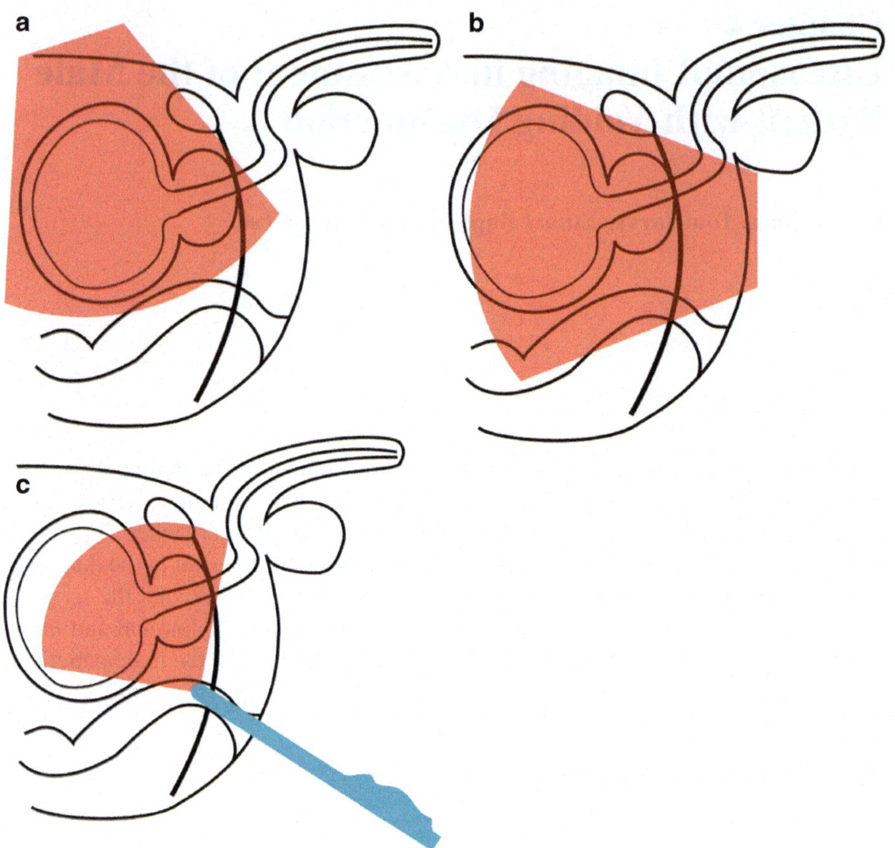

Fig. 4.1 (**a**) Transabdominal ultrasound scan of pelvis. (**b**) Transperineal ultrasound scan. (**c**) Transrectal ultrasound scan (intracavity transducer)

Technique of Transabdominal Ultrasound

The examination is easily performed using 2D ultrasound equipment and a curved transducer for abdominal scanning (for example, a 2–5 MHz transducer). It is important to identify the pubic symphysis and place the transducer above this level and angulate the transducer appropriately to avoid loss of field of view caused by shadowing behind the pubic bone (Fig. 4.2). Common measurements in the male patient with voiding dysfunction include pre and post void residual volumes (Fig. 4.3), prostate volume (Fig. 4.4), bladder wall thickness and intravesical prostatic protrusion (Fig. 4.5). The scanning technique is detailed in Tips 4.1.

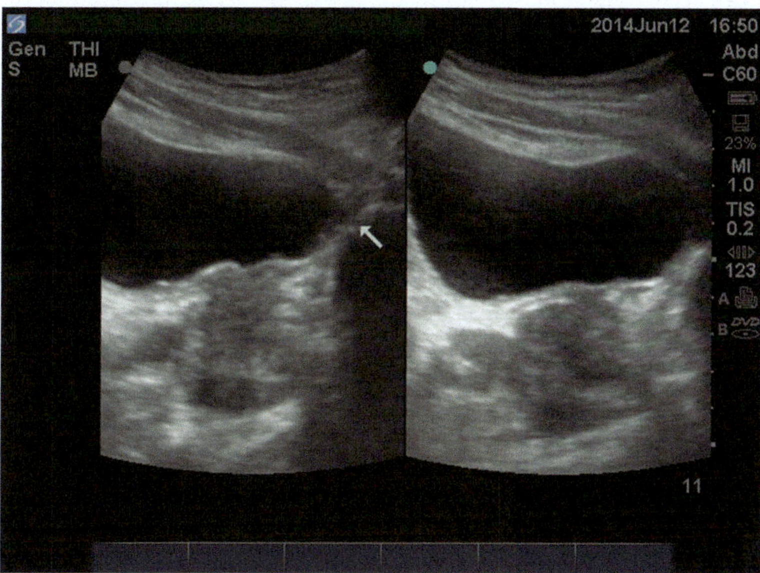

Fig. 4.2 Transabdominal ultrasound image of male pelvis (sagittal plane). It is important to identify the pubic symphysis and angulate the transducer appropriately to avoid loss of view caused by acoustic shadowing behind the pubic bone (*arrow*)

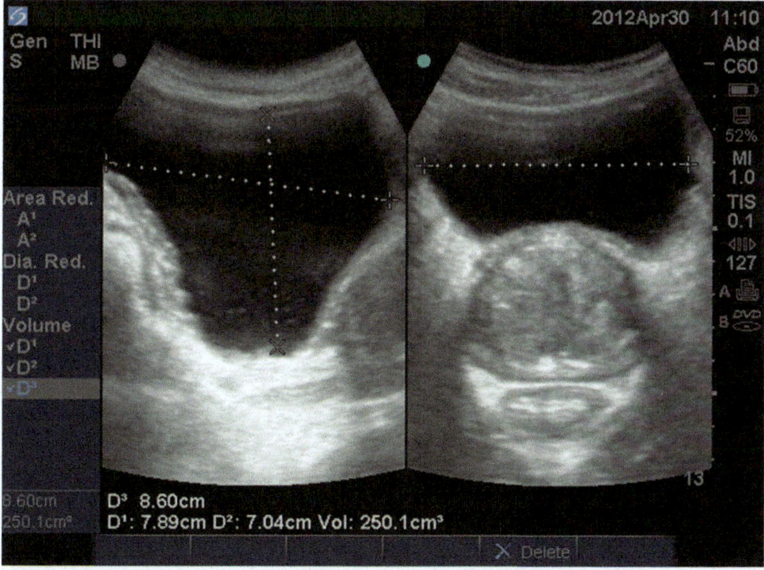

Fig. 4.3 Postvoid residual urine volume measurement. Ultrasound images of bladder in sagittal and transverse planes showing elevated residual urine and prostatomegaly

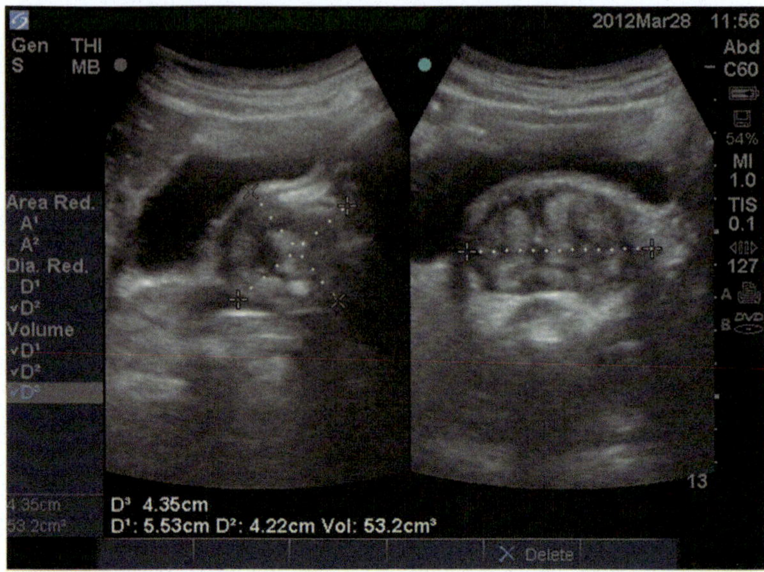

Fig. 4.4 Prostate volume measurement. Transabdominal ultrasound images of prostate in sagittal (*left* image) and transverse planes (*right* image)

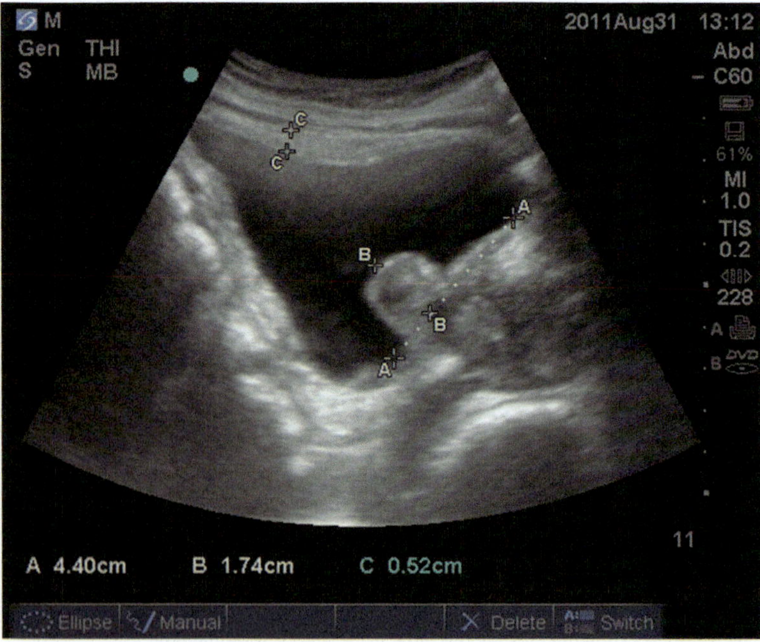

Fig. 4.5 Measurement of intravesical prostatic protrusion (*B*) as a perpendicular line from the bladder base (*A*), and bladder wall thickness (*C*)

Tips 4.1 Easy Steps to Performing Bladder Ultrasound
(a) Image with the patient supine
(b) Palpate pubic symphysis and place transducer above this level for scanning
(c) Start scan in sagittal plane
(d) Identify bladder, bladder neck and prostate
(e) Adjust depth of field and focus (see Figs. 2.7 and 2.16)
(f) Movement of transducer (sweeping/sliding/'rocking' movements) to cover the entire bladder in sagittal plane
(g) Change to transverse plane

Transperineal Ultrasound

The male pelvis can also be imaged via the perineum. This approach (Fig. 4.6) has an emerging role in the evaluation of the pelvic floor in post-prostatectomy incontinence (see Cases 2 and 3). It also provides satisfactory imaging of the prostate for the measurement of prostate volume (which may be more acceptable than a transrectal route) given the difficulty in imaging the apex of the prostate for accurate volume measurement by the transabdominal route [1]. Transperineal ultrasound can also be used to image the prostate to guide biopsies in patients

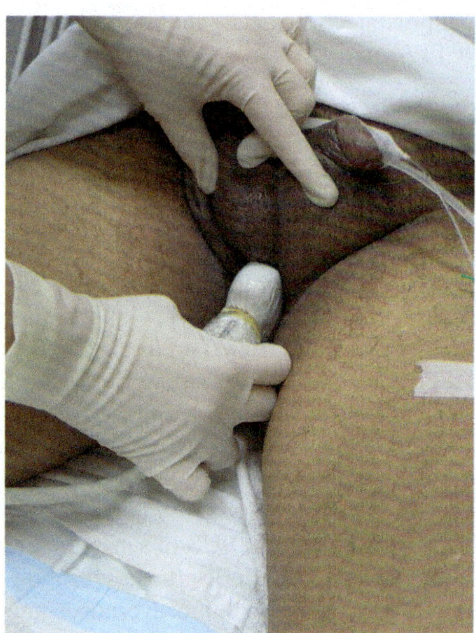

Fig. 4.6 Transducer placement for transperineal ultrasound in the male patient. The scrotum is lifted cephalad to allow placement of the transducer against the perineum

Tips 4.2 Technique of Transperineal Imaging of the Male Pelvic Floor
(a) Image with the patient supine with legs slightly flexed and abducted
(b) Lift scrotum cephaled to expose perineum
(c) Scan in sagittal plane (Fig. 4.13)
(d) Identify pubic symphysis, bladder, bladder neck and bulbar urethra
(e) Adjust depth of field and focus
(f) Identify sling (if present) in mid-sagittal plane, avoiding excessive pressure on the perineum which may distort anatomy
(g) Assessment of movement of sling, compression of urethra during valsalva/cough (video)
(h) Assess pelvic floor contraction

who have undergone abdominal-perineal (AP) excision of the rectum and thus are unable to have transrectal ultrasound. The scanning technique is detailed in Tips 4.2.

Applications of Pelvic Floor Ultrasound in Physiotherapy

Two useful applications for ultrasound imaging in the physiotherapy management of the urological patient are for stress urinary incontinence (SUI) post radical prostatectomy (RP) and in men presenting with chronic pelvic pain syndrome (CPPS).

Stress Urinary Incontinence (SUI)

Pelvic floor muscle strengthening has long been advocated for men as an intervention aimed at improving continence recovery post RP. Transperineal ultrasound gives a very clear field of view of the Anorectal junction (ARJ), Bulbar penile crus, and urethra. The striated urethral sphincter (SUS) can also be viewed (Fig. 4.7)

Prior to any kind of strength training accurate isolation of the correct muscles must first be achieved. Our aim is to reduce the dominant posterior levator ani action (anal component) of the pelvic floor contraction and instead educate the patient on a more anterior penile and SUS lift sensation.

Verbal cues are given to elicit less anterosuperior motion at the ARJ and more posterior slide of the SUS (a sensation of testicular vertical lifting) and an anterior slide of the bulbar penile crus (a sensation of penile indrawing – as if ceasing urination produced by the bulbocavernosus muscle).

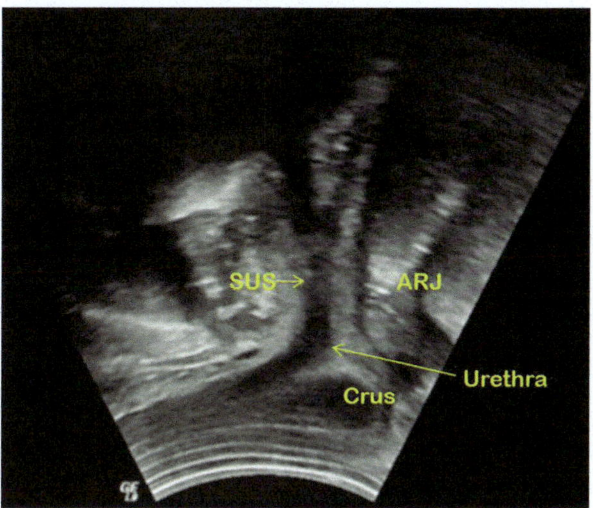

Fig. 4.7 Transperineal ultrasound imaging for pelvic floor muscle strengthening feedback

The combination of posterior SUS motion and anterior bulbocavernosus contraction causes increasing urethral closure pressure and is therefore considered to be vital in improving continence outcomes [8].

Once evidence of high quality motor control is observed on ultrasound using verbal cueing then the patient may be encouraged to continue with a progressive hypertrophy program designed to further increase urethral closure pressure under progressive loads and functional movement patterns.

Male Chronic Pelvic Pain Syndrome (CPPS)

Also called Chronic Prostatitis, Proctalgia Fugax and Pudendal Neuraligia (amongst other names) this painful condition can often baffle the most experienced clinicians as there is often very little clinical evidence of an organic dysfunction. Cystoscopy, urinalysis, urodynamic and blood tests are often all within normal limits. The patient is often frustrated and frightened and is almost always in a state of high stress and anxiety.

Often the only clinical feature is an abnormally high anal sphincter tone and excessive discomfort during digital rectal examination (even though the prostatic tissue may feel within normal limits).

In these cases pelvic floor hypertonicity may be a contributing and perpetuating factor in this disabling condition.

Transabdominal ultrasound scanning can be a useful tool in evaluating bladder base rise/fall on contraction and release of pelvic floor contractions. Hypertonicity

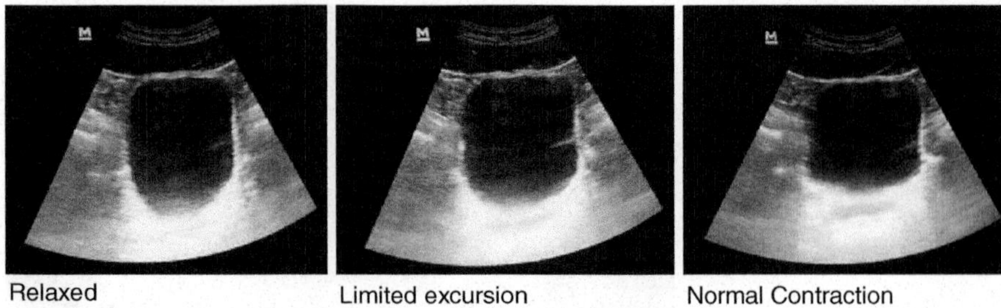

Fig. 4.8 Ultrasound of bladder base rise/fall on contraction and release of pelvic floor muscles

can be seen as a poor bladder base rise on volitional pelvic floor muscle activation and a slow return to a more rested/relaxed state following cessation of pelvic floor muscle activity (Fig. 4.8).

Relaxation of the pelvic floor musclulature can be taught whilst observing the bladder base during respiration. Hypertonic pelvic floors have a tendancy to prevent bladder base descent during inspiration. By giving patients cues to 'release tension' in the pelvic floor during the inspiratory phase of respiration (as intra-abdominal pressure increases) increased excursion of the bladder base in a caudad direction may be observed on ultrasound.

Continued practice of effective pelvic floor relaxation may be crucial in assisting in restoring normal pelvic floor tone to the patient with CPPS.

Cases

The following cases illustrate applications of pelvic floor ultrasound in assessment of the male patient with voiding dysfunction.

Case 1 Voiding Dysfunction

A 65-year-old man presented with reduced urinary flow, frequency, nocturia and a sensation of incomplete bladder emptying (Fig. 4.5, Video 4.1).

Comments

The images demonstrate prominent intra-vesical protrusion of the prostate. Various ultrasound imaging parameters have been investigated for the evaluation of bladder outlet obstruction in addition to functional parameters such as uroflow and pressure-flow urodynamic studies. These ultrasound measurements include prostate

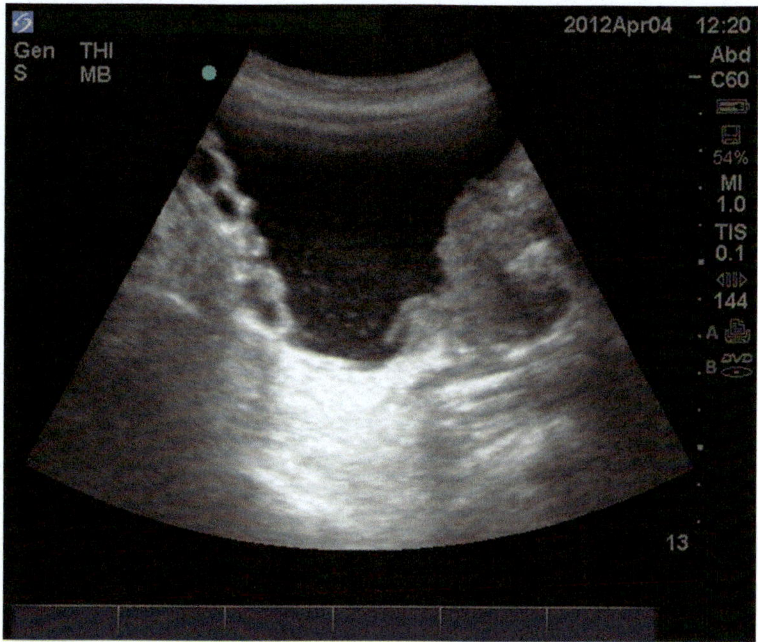

Fig. 4.9 Trabeculation of bladder wall with saccules in a male patient with chronic bladder outlet obstruction

volume, post-void residual (PVR) urine measurement, bladder wall thickness and measurement of intravesical protrusion of the prostate. Prostate volume and residual urine has poor correlation with urodynamic outlet obstruction and the role of bladder wall thickness is controversial [2, 3]. Of all these parameters, the degree of intravesical protrusion of the prostate (Fig. 4.5) appears to have the best correlation with outlet obstruction [4].

Other ultrasound features of bladder outlet obstruction include trabeculation (Fig. 4.9), the presence of bladder diverticulum (Fig. 4.10) and presence of bladder calculi. Bladder calculi can generally be distinguished from calcified bladder tumours by tilting the patient and re-imaging in the decubitus position as calculi are mobile within the bladder (Fig. 4.11).

Ultrasound can also be employed as the imaging modality for urodynamic studies in certain circumstances. Transabdominal imaging during the filling phase of urodynamics allows detection of bladder trabeculation, intravesical prostatic protrusion and upper urinary tract assessment. Upper urinary tract dilatation may indicate effect of outlet obstruction or reflux (Fig. 4.12). However, it is generally not possible to image the urethra during voiding. A protocol for ultrasound imaging during urodynamic study is included in Tips 4.3.

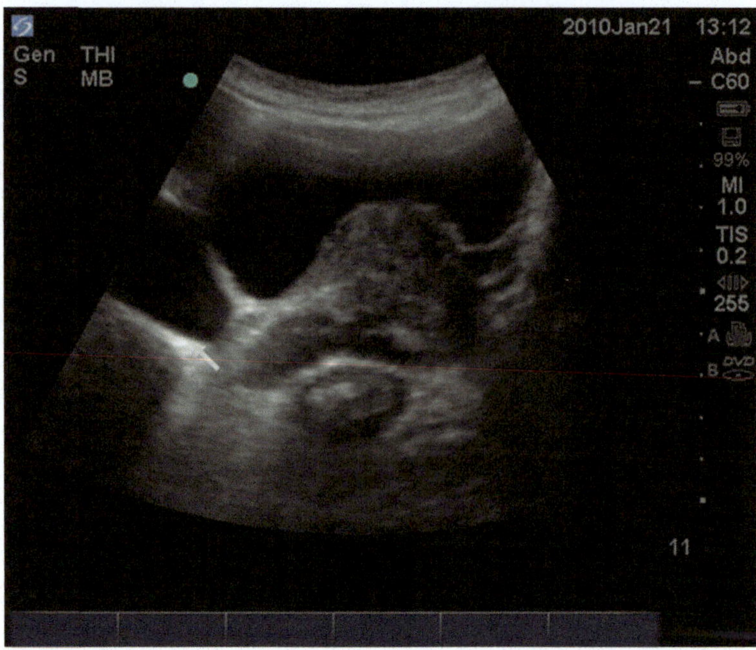

Fig. 4.10 Bladder diverticulum. Transverse image of the bladder in a male patient with bladder outlet obstruction and a right sided bladder diverticulum (*arrow*)

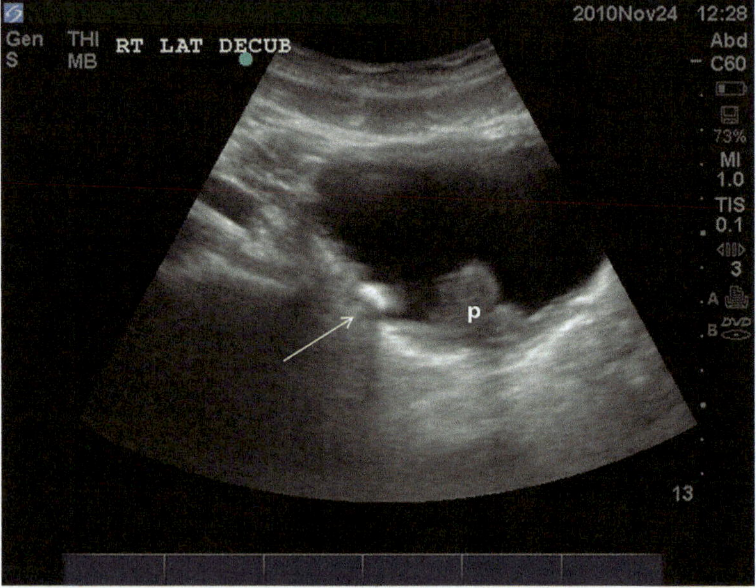

Fig. 4.11 Bladder calculus. Decubitus image of bladder demonstrating echogenic calculus (*arrow*) with posterior acoustic shadowing. Prostate (*p*)

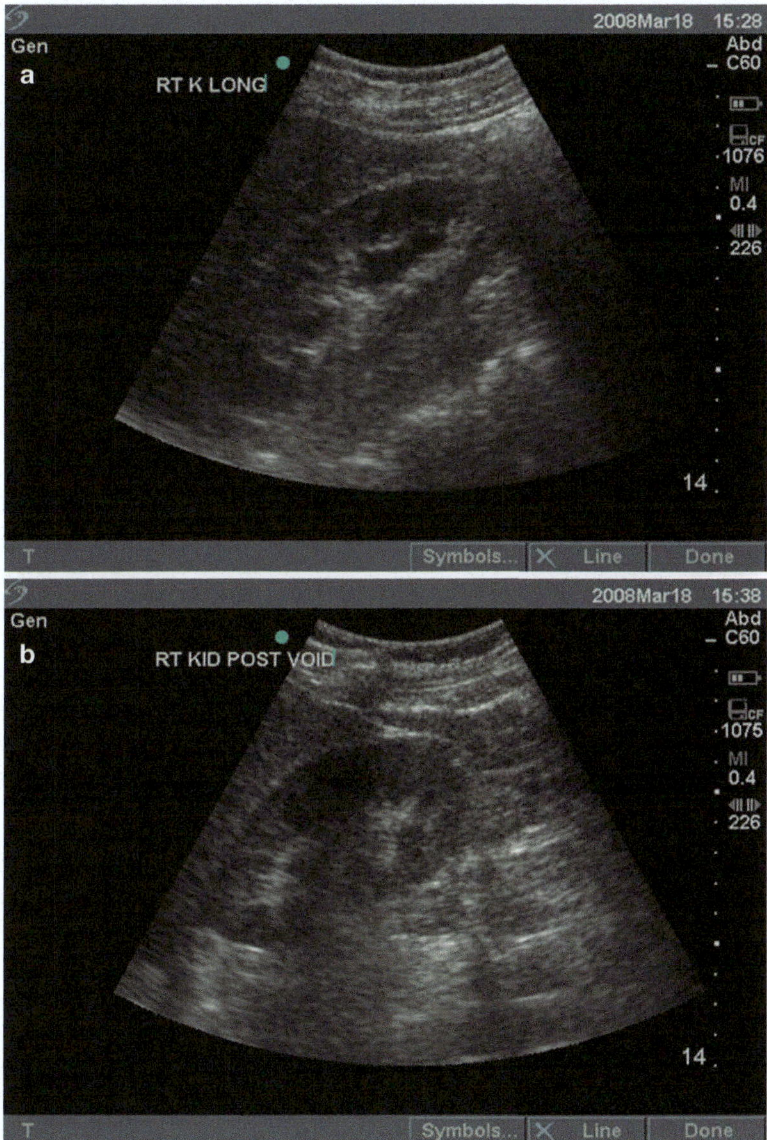

Fig. 4.12 (**a**) Sagittal image of kidney (obtained during ultrasound urodynamics) in a patient with bladder outlet obstruction and reduced detrusor compliance demonstrating dilatation of collecting system during bladder filling. The hydronephrosis resolved post voiding (**b**)

Tips 4.3 Imaging Protocol for Ultrasound Urodynamics in Males

(a) Imaging of bladder at beginning of filling phase to confirm catheter position if necessary
(b) Bladder/prostate imaging at filling volume of 150 ml (anterior bladder wall thickness measured on mid sagittal plane and intravesical protrusion of prostate)
(c) Upper tract imaging (hydronephrosis/calculi) especially in neurogenic bladder patients
(d) Repeat bladder imaging +/– upper tract imaging at or near capacity
(e) Postvoid residual measurement at end of urodynamics

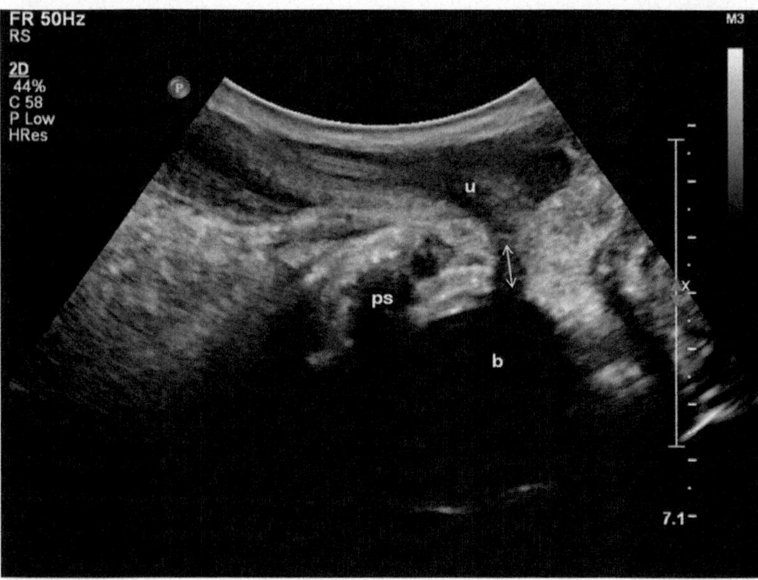

Fig. 4.13 Sagittal transperineal ultrasound image of patient with urinary incontinence post radical prostatectomy. Bladder (*b*), pubic symphysis (*ps*), urethra (bulbar) (*u*), external sphincter (*arrow*)

Case 2 Post Prostatectomy Incontinence

A 65-year-old male presented with persisting severe urinary incontinence 18 months after a radical prostatectomy. He has tried pelvic floor (Kegel) exercises with little improvement (Fig. 4.13 and Video 4.2).

Comments Pelvic floor ultrasound in the assessment of post-prostatectomy incontinence

Although urge incontinence is the most common type of incontinence in men and usually occurs in the setting of an overactive bladder, stress incontinence may occur following prostate surgery and is of increasing importance due to the popularity of radical prostatectomy as treatment for prostate cancer.

Urinary incontinence occurring after radical prostatectomy has a reported incidence of 2–60 % with a median of 10–15 %. The reported rates vary according to the definition of incontinence and the methods of evaluation (such as questionnaires, interviews by clinician vs independent reviewer). Risk factors identified include advanced age, stage of disease and previous radiation therapy. The surgical approach to radical prostatectomy (retropubic, perineal, laparoscopic/robotic) does not appear to be a significant factor [5].

Urodynamic evaluation is important to identify the underlying pathophysiology in patients with post- prostatectomy incontinence prior to consideration of surgical treatment. Although sphincteric incompetence/deficiency is the main cause of the incontinence in more than two thirds of patients, detrusor overactivity or poor compliance may be present in 40–60 % [6]. With an increasing number of treatment options for mild to moderate stress incontinence available, identification and management of associated detrusor dysfunction may therefore influence the ultimate choice of surgical treatment.

Transperineal ultrasound may be used as an alternative mode of imaging during urodynamics and can replace fluoroscopy. Dynamic transperineal 2D imaging allows assessment of the bladder, bladder neck beaking (Video 4.2) and urethral mobility. The clinician can also assess pelvic floor contractions and the success of a pelvic floor muscle (Kegel) exercise program which is commonly prescribed for patients with post prostatectomy incontinence (Video 4.3). MRI and ultrasound studies have shown that there is little urethral mobility/hypermobility in patients with post prostatectomy incontinence (unlike female stress incontinence) [7], (Fig. 4.14) so it is acceptable to perform perineal ultrasound with the patient lying comfortably in a supine position with legs slightly flexed and abducted (Fig. 4.6)- see Tips 4.2.

It is easier to assess bladder, bladder neck and urethral morphology during dynamic scanning with some urine in the bladder (ideally more than 100–150 ml). In practice, however, many patients with severe incontinence void frequently to reduce bladder volume and hence amount of stress incontinence. They may be unable to retain significant amount of urine for ultrasound assessment (video 4.2).

In trouble-shooting patients with a urinary prosthesis such as artificial urinary sphincter, ultrasound is useful to measure volume of fluid in the reservoir to detect leakage of fluid from the system (Fig. 4.15).

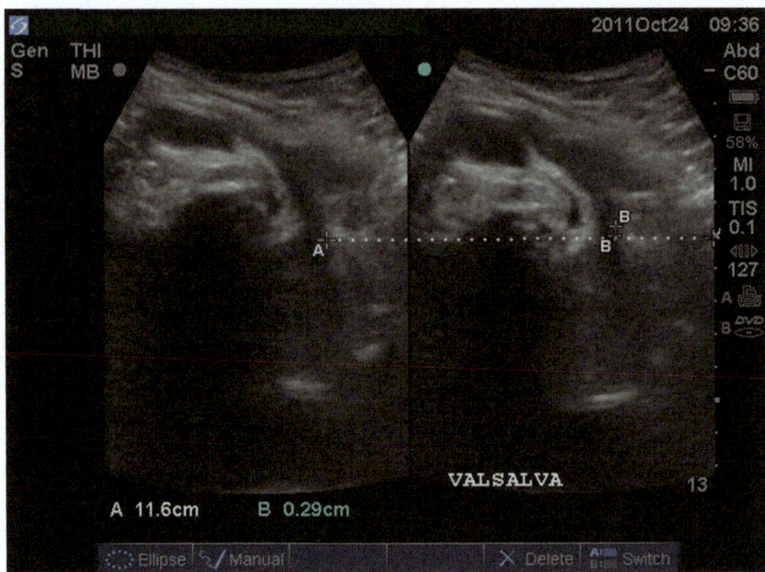

Fig. 4.14 Transperineal ultrasound images of patient with urinary incontinence post radical prostatectomy, at rest (*left*) and on Valsalva (*right*) demonstrating minimal urethral descent (*B*). The urethrovesical anastomosis/bladder neck at rest (*A*)

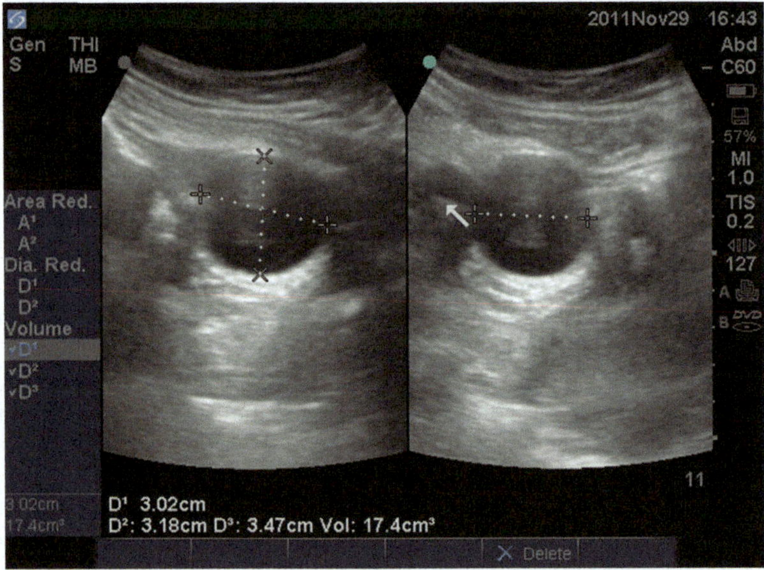

Fig. 4.15 Transabdominal ultrasound image of the pressure regulating balloon of an artificial urinary sphincter (AMS 800). The *arrow* indicates position of the tubing

Case 3 Post Prostatectomy Incontinence: Failed Male Sling

A 67-year-old male who underwent transobturator synthetic sling for incontinence post radical retropubic prostatectomy still requires the use of three medium pads per day. Preoperative urodynamic studies showed normal bladder capacity and a 24-h pad weight was 400 g. The patient reported initial improvement post-operatively but had significant deterioration in his continence at 3 weeks. Transperineal ultrasound scan was performed to assess sling position in this patient with early sling failure (Video 4.5).

Comments Dynamic scanning: The evolving role of transperineal ultrasound in evaluation of male slings

There has been increasing use of transobturator slings in the treatment of post-prostatectomy stress urinary incontinence (Fig. 4.16). Three year data demonstrates these slings to be safe and effective in mild to moderate post-prostatectomy incontinence [8]. Whilst the exact mechanism of action of these slings remains unclear, transperineal ultrasound studies of male slings have demonstrated the phenomenon of 'dynamic compression' of the urethra (Fig. 4.17a, b, Video 4.4) with coughing and Valsalva that may be a mechanism of action apart from direct compression of the urethra. As synthetic slings are easily visualised on ultrasound, there is an evolving role in the use of dynamic transperineal ultrasound imaging to evaluate patients with failed slings (also see Tips 4.2)

In this patient the transperineal ultrasound images (Fig. 4.18, Video 4.5) showed that there was displacement/malposition of the sling causing early sling failure. The patient subsequently had a successful re-do sling procedure (Fig. 4.19).

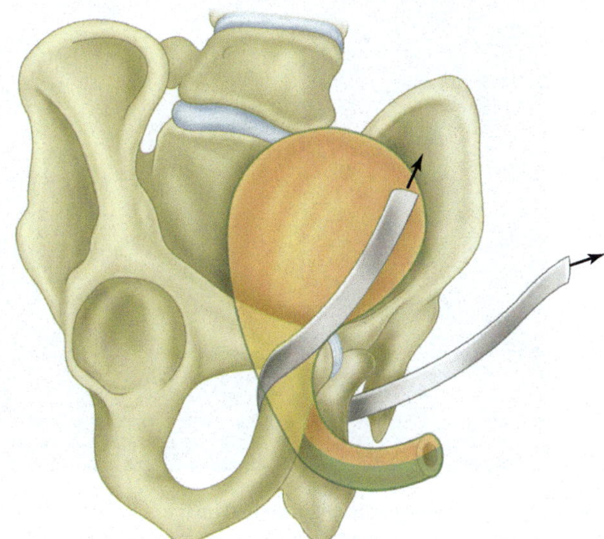

Fig. 4.16 Male trans-obturator sling (Advance sling- image courtesy of American Medical Systems)

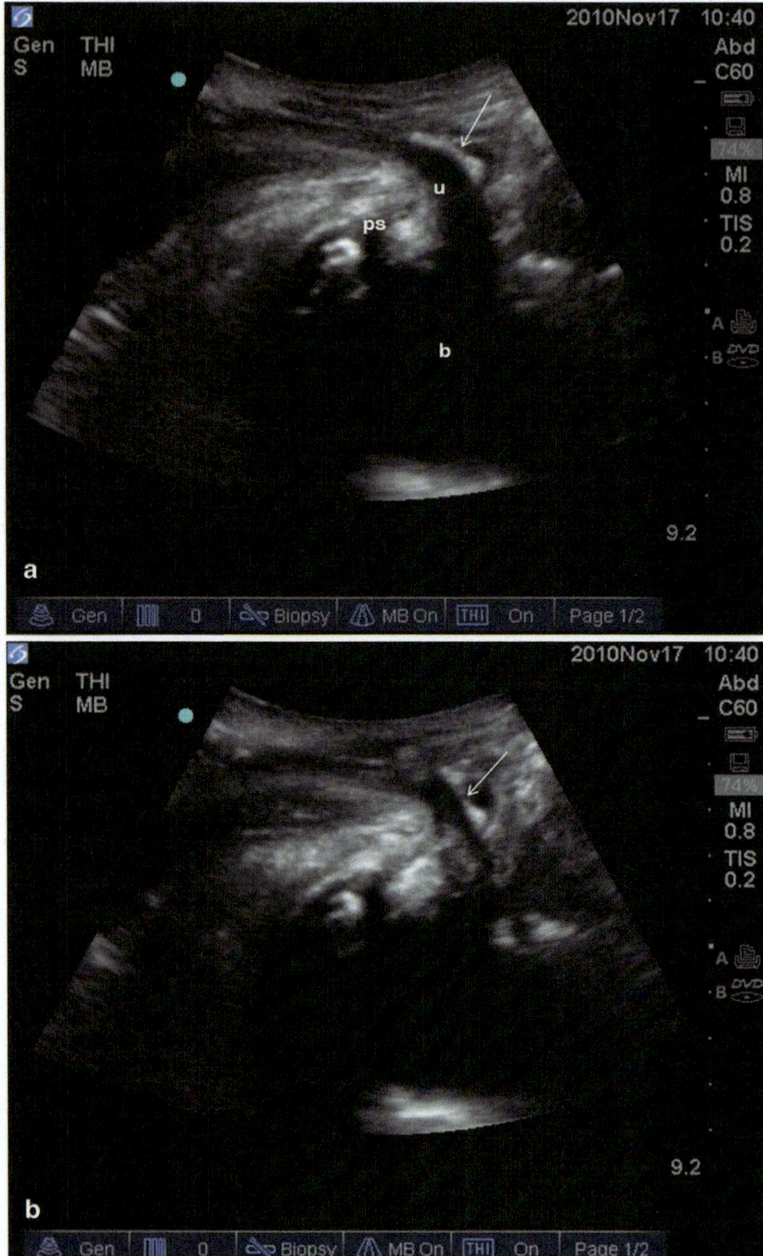

Fig. 4.17 Sagittal transperineal ultrasound images of AdVance sling at rest (**a**) and on coughing (**b**) demonstrating dynamic compression of the urethra. Bladder (*b*), pubic symphysis (*ps*), urethra (bulbar) (*u*), sling (*arrow*)

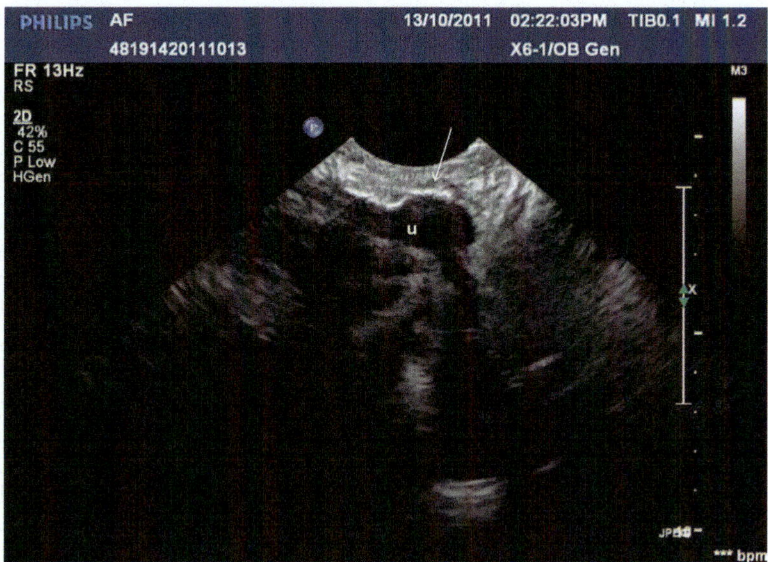

Fig. 4.18 Transperineal ultrasound image during Valsalva in patient with early failure post Advance sling showing malposition and lack of urethral compression *(arrow)*. Urethra (bulbar) (*u*)

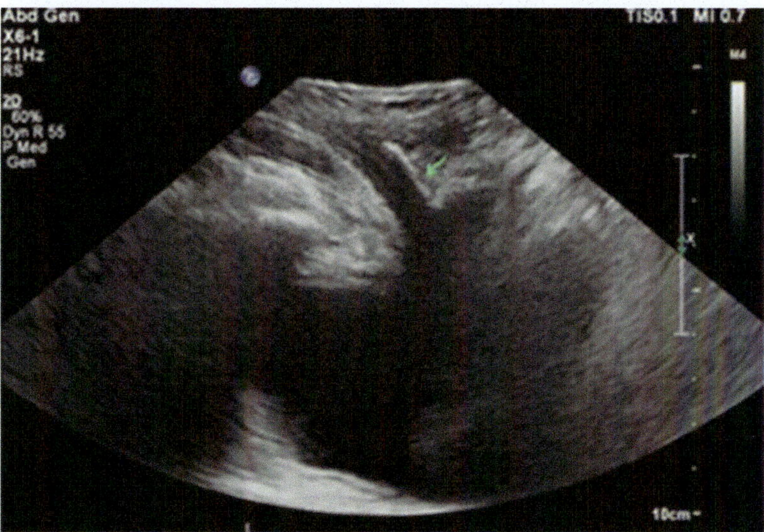

Fig. 4.19 Transperineal ultrasound image in patient who underwent re-do AdVance XP sling (green arrow) following early failure due to malpositioning

References

1. Griffiths KA, Ly LP, Jin B, Chan L, Handelsman DJ. Transperineal ultrasound for measurement of prostate volume: validation against transrectal ultrasound. J Urol. 2007;178(4 Pt1): 1375–9.
2. Blatt AH, Titus J, Chan L. Ultrasound measurement of bladder wall thickness in the assessment of voiding dysfunction. J Urol. 2008;179(6):2275–8.
3. Franco G, De Nunzio C, Constantino L, Tubaro A, Ciccarello M. Ultrasound assessment of intravesical prostatic protrusion and detrusor wall thickness – new standards for noninvasive bladder outlet obstruction diagnosis? J Urol. 2010;183:2270–4.
4. Chia SJ, Heng CT, Chan SP, Foo KT. Correlation of intravesical prostatic protrusion with bladder outlet obstruction. BJU Int. 2003;914(4):371–4.
5. Herschorn S, Thuroff J, Bruschini H, Grise P, Hanus T, Kakizaki H, Kirschner-Hermanns R, Nitti V, Schick E. Surgical treatment of urinary incontinence in men. In: Incontinence Proceedings of the 3rd International Consultation on Incontinence, vol 2. Paris: Health Publication Ltd; 2005. p. 1241–96.
6. Groutz A, Blaivas J, Chaikin D, Weiss J, Verhaaren M. The pathophysiology of post-radical prostatectomy incontinence: a clinical and video urodynamics study. J Urol. 2000;163(6): 1767–70.
7. Suskind AM, DeLancey JO, Hussain HK, Montgomery JS, Latini JM, Cameron AP. Dynamic MRI evaluation of urethral hypermobility post- radical prostatectomy. NeurourolUrodyn. 2014;33:312–5.
8. Stafford RE, Ashton-Miller JA, Constantinou CE, Hodges PW. A new method to quantify male pelvic floor displacement from 2D transperineal ultrasound images. Urology. 2013;81(3): 685–9.

Chapter 5
Pelvic Ultrasound in the Assessment of Female Voiding Dysfunction

Lewis Chan

The female pelvis can be imaged via transabdominal, transperineal and transvaginal approaches. There is little doubt that transvaginal imaging is the technique of choice for imaging of the pelvic organs; this is covered in Chap. 7.

Transabdominal imaging is often the initial modality of imaging in assessment of patients with voiding dysfunction. A pelvic ultrasound scan performed via the transabdominal route (Fig. 5.1) allows easy assessment of the bladder, post-void residual (PVR) urine measurements, identification of ureteric jets and general survey of female pelvic organs. There is also a role in the assessment of upper urinary tract especially in cases of voiding dysfunction or suspected neurogenic bladder.

However, in the assessment of voiding dysfunction, urinary incontinence and pelvic organ prolapse, the transperineal approach (Fig. 5.2) allows for an easy, non-invasive method of imaging the three compartments of the pelvic floor. Furthermore, there is little distortion of anatomy and patient discomfort because the transducer is placed externally. Transperineal imaging is often conducted with the patient in supine position (Fig. 5.3) but the standing position (Fig. 5.4) can be utilized and is useful for the assessment of incontinence and pelvic organ prolapse.

Slings and synthetic meshes are easily visible as echogenic structures on ultrasound and transperineal imaging allows for good assessment especially in patients with a failed sling or complications post sling.

For most patients with voiding dysfunction, incontinence and pelvic organ prolapse, 2D imaging is sufficient but 3D imaging has an emerging role in evaluation of prolapse and meshes (see Chaps. 6 and 9).

Electronic supplementary material The online version of this chapter (doi: 10.1007/978-3-319-04310-4_5) contains supplementary material, which is available to authorized users.

L. Chan, MBBS(Hons), FRACS, DDU
Department of Urology, Concord Repatriation General Hospital, Sydney, NSW, Australia
e-mail: lewis.chan@sswahs.nsw.gov.au

L. Chan et al. (eds.), *Pelvic Floor Ultrasound: Principles, Applications and Case Studies*, DOI 10.1007/978-3-319-04310-4_5

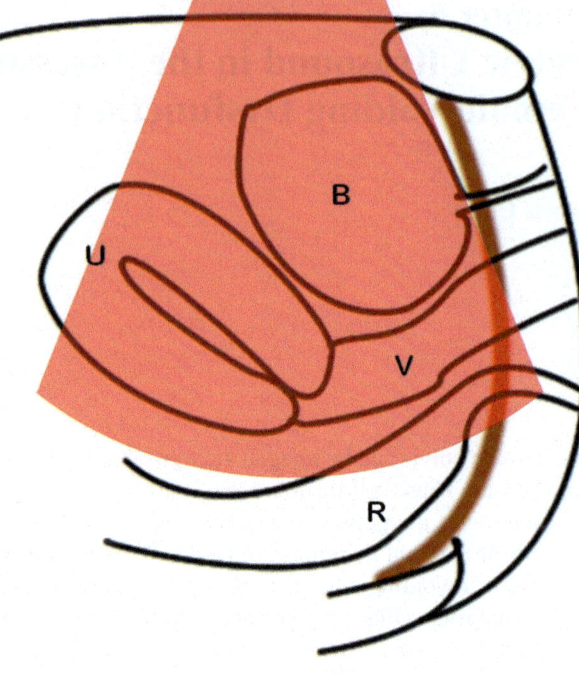

Fig. 5.1 Transabdominal ultrasound of the pelvis (*B* bladder, *V* vagina, *U* uterus, *R* rectum)

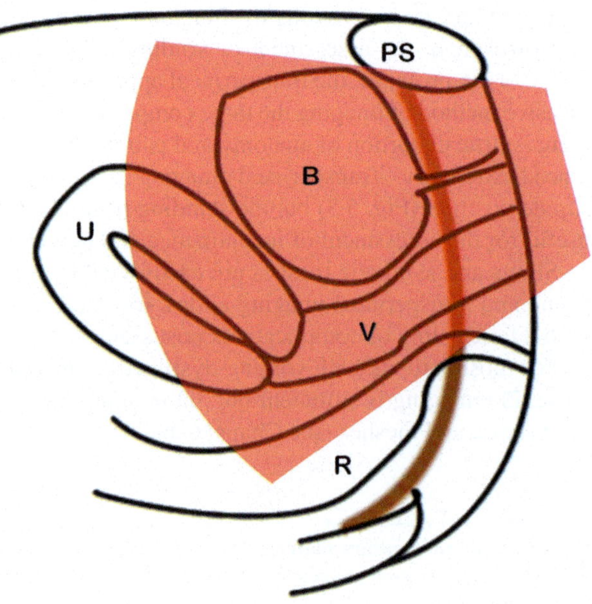

Fig. 5.2 Transperineal ultrasound of the pelvis (*B* bladder, *V* vagina, *U* uterus, *R* rectum, *PS* pubic symphysis)

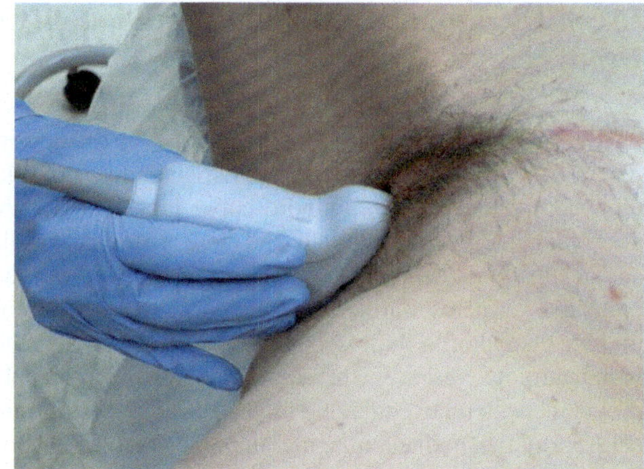

Fig. 5.3 Transducer placement for transperineal (translabial) ultrasound

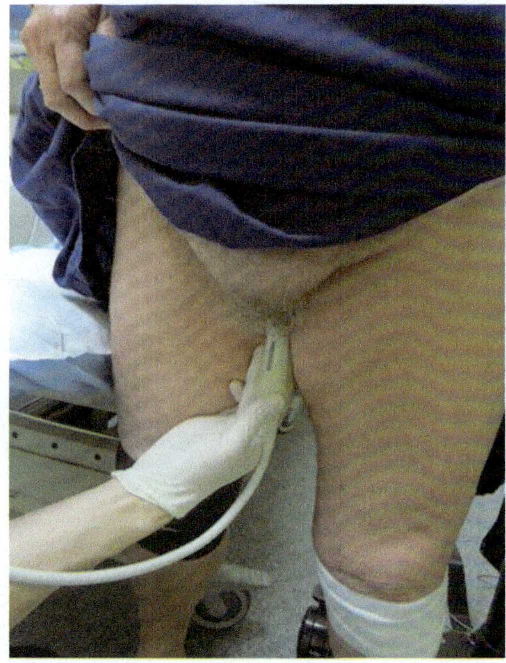

Fig. 5.4 Transducer placement for transperineal (translabial) ultrasound with the patient standing

Use of Ultrasound as the Imaging Modality for Video Urodynamics

Urodynamics are a commonly performed investigation in the evaluation of patients with voiding dysfunction and arguably remain the 'gold standard'. Traditionally video urodynamics have utilized fluoroscopic imaging. However, not all clinicians have access to radiological equipment and there is the risk of radiation exposure to the patient and occupational exposure to the clinician, as well as the requirement to wear heavy protective garments. Furthermore, depending on the equipment, the patient may have to transfer on and off a fluoroscopy table. This poses difficulty for the elderly or patients with neurologic disease. Ultrasound imaging (by suprapubic and transperineal routes) provides an alternative imaging modality of the lower urinary tract during urodynamics (Fig. 5.5). Transperineal imaging, in particular, allows good visualization of the pelvic floor and arguably provides more information than contrast fluoroscopy in assessment of urinary incontinence and pelvic organ prolapse. This is especially the case if there is mesh or a sling present as these are easily visible on ultrasound. A protocol for using ultrasound as the imaging modality for urodynamics is attached (Tips 5.1).

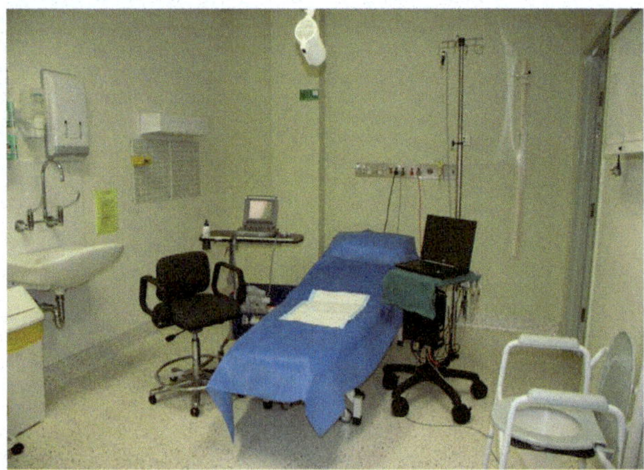

Fig. 5.5 Room setup for video-urodynamics utilising ultrasound imaging (also see Chap. 3)

Tips 5.1 Imaging Protocol for Ultrasound Urodynamics in the Female Patient

(a) Transabdominal imaging of bladder at beginning of filling phase to confirm catheter position if necessary
(b) Bladder imaging at filling volume of 150 ml
(c) Upper tract imaging (hydronephrosis/calculi) especially in neurogenic bladder patients
(d) Repeat bladder imaging +/− upper tract imaging at or near capacity (to identify reflux)
(e) Dynamic translabial imaging (bladder neck/urethra/ POP) performed with patient standing after removal of filling catheter, at rest and on Valsalva/cough

(f) Bladder neck descent/mobility measured relative to inferior aspect of pubic symphysis in mid sagittal plane
(g) Assessment of pelvic floor contraction
(h) Post-void residual measurement at end of urodynamics

A Technique of Transperineal 2D Imaging (Tips 5.2)

Indications

Assessment of urinary incontinence, pelvic organ prolapse, and slings/mesh complications.

Equipment

Transperineal (translabial) 2D ultrasound can be performed using standard gray-scale ultrasound equipment and the curved array transducer (e.g. 2–5 MHz) used for transabdominal imaging.

Transducer Placement

The transducer is placed on perineum in the sagittal plane (Fig. 5.3) and the image can be orientated according to the preference of the clinician (Videos 5.1 and 5.2). The key anatomic landmarks are pubic symphysis, urethra, bladder, vagina and rectum (Figs. 5.2 and 5.6).

Scanning Position

Patient can be scanned in the supine or standing positions. It is important to avoid excessive pressure of the transducer against the perineum that may cause discomfort and/or distort anatomy.

Movements of the Transducer

The 'rocking' manoeuver allows the field of view to be adjusted covering the compartment of interest (anterior, middle or posterior). It is important to adjust the depth-of-view setting to the region of interest.

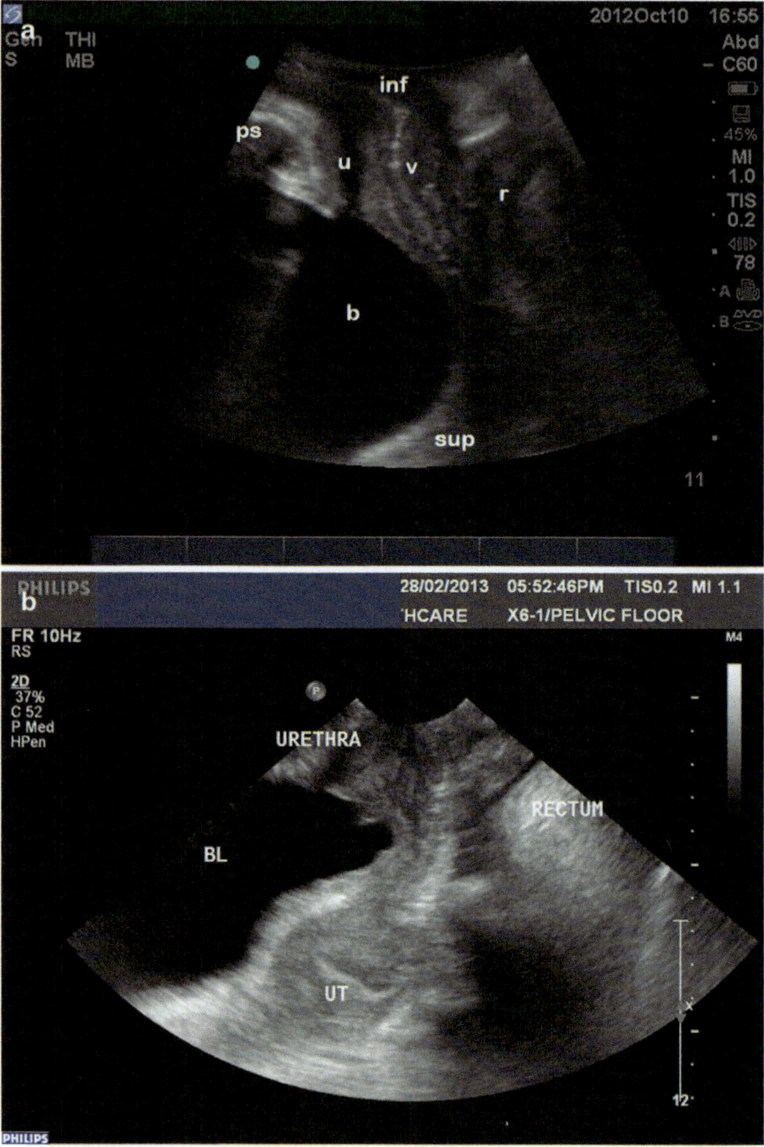

Fig. 5.6 (**a**, **b**) Sagittal transperineal ultrasound images demonstrating the three compartments of the pelvis. Bladder (*b*), urethra (*u*), vagina (*v*), rectum (*r*), pubic symphysis (*ps*), inferior/caudal (*inf*), superior/cranial (*sup*), *UT* uterus

Dynamic Imaging

The ability of ultrasound to obtain dynamic imaging information is an important advantage of this modality of imaging in the assessment of the pelvic floor. This should be tailored to the clinical problem, hence the importance of clinician input in performance of scans.

Dynamic assessment during transperineal ultrasound include evaluation of the bladder neck and urethral mobility, pelvic organ prolapse during Valsalva and cough, as well as pelvic floor contractions (Video 5.3). Some of these may be best performed with the patient in the standing position (Fig. 5.4). Dynamic imaging can be incorporated as part of video-urodynamics (see Case 1).

Pelvic floor ultrasound can also be used as an adjunct for pelvic floor physiotherapy. This can be performed via transabdominal or transperineal approaches and is usually performed with some urine in bladder (e.g. about 1–200 ml) but not overfilled. Dynamic 2D imaging can detect pelvic floor contraction/'lift' (see Video 5.4).

Tips 5.2 Tips for Transperineal Imaging

(a) Use adequate gel to ensure good transducer coupling
(b) Start scan in sagittal plane (Fig. 5.6)
(c) Identify bladder, urethra, vagina and rectum
(d) Adjust depth of field and focus
(e) Movement of transducer by rocking to capture desired field of view (i.e. anterior/middle/posterior compartments)
(f) Ask patient to cough, Valsalva and contract their pelvic floor for dynamic assessment

Clinical Cases

The following cases illustrate the utility of 2D pelvic ultrasound in the assessment of voiding dysfunction.

Case 1: Stress Urinary Incontinence

A 50-year-old female presented with symptoms of stress urinary incontinence requiring the use of two pads a day, especially when she exercised (Video 5.5 and Fig. 5.7). Stress incontinence was demonstrated during urodynamics.

Comments These transperineal ultrasound images (and video captured during urodynamic study) show rotational descent with beaking and opening of the bladder neck during Valsalva and cough consistent with urethral hypermobility. This is commonly treated with placement of a mid urethral sling [1].

In the ultrasound assessment of incontinence it is often useful to perform the scan with the patient in the standing position and with at least 200 ml in the bladder to reproduce the exact situation and anatomic configuration when the patient usually experiences stress incontinence (Fig. 5.4).

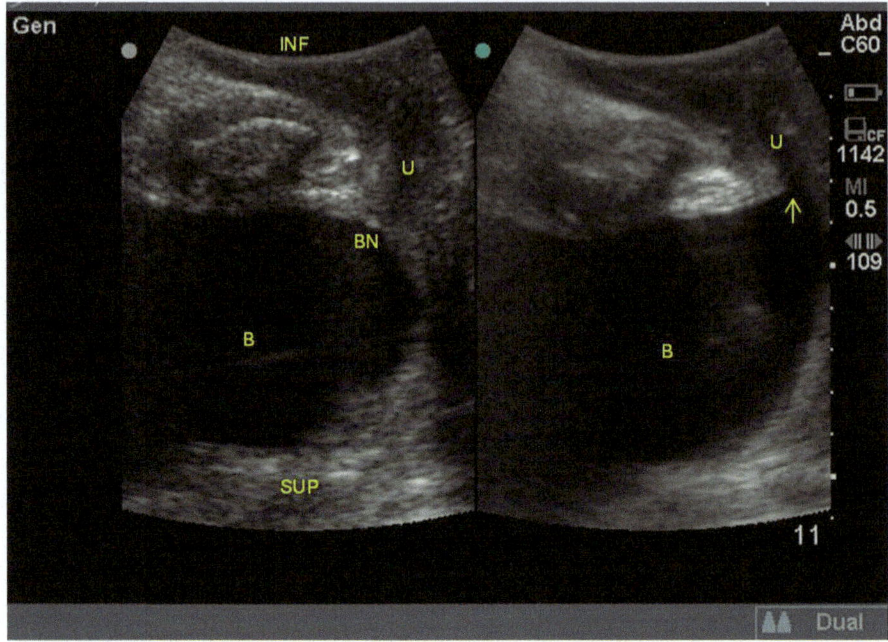

Fig. 5.7 Urethral hypermobility – Transperineal ultrasound image of bladder (*B*) and urethra (*U*) at rest (*left image*) and with straining (*right image*) demonstrating rotational descent of the urethra with opening of the bladder neck/proximal urethra (*arrow*) leading to stress incontinence. *BN* bladder neck, *INF* inferior /caudal, *SUP* superior/cranial

Case 2: Severe Urinary Incontinence

An 80-year-old female presented with severe urinary incontinence during any activity. There was no pelvic organ prolapse on clinical examination. She requires the use of pull-up pants.

Comments The images (Fig. 5.8) demonstrate an open bladder neck with little descent with cough or Valsalva. This finding is consistent with intrinsic urethral sphincter deficiency. Such patients have poorer results with mid-urethral synthetic slings and may be considered for a pubo-vaginal fascial sling or injection of a urethral bulking agent.

Case 3: Persisting Incontinence Post Sling Procedure

A 70-year-old female with presented with persisting stress urinary incontinence following a transobturator sling procedure. She underwent urodynamic study with transperineal ultrasound imaging (Fig 5.9 and Video 5.6).

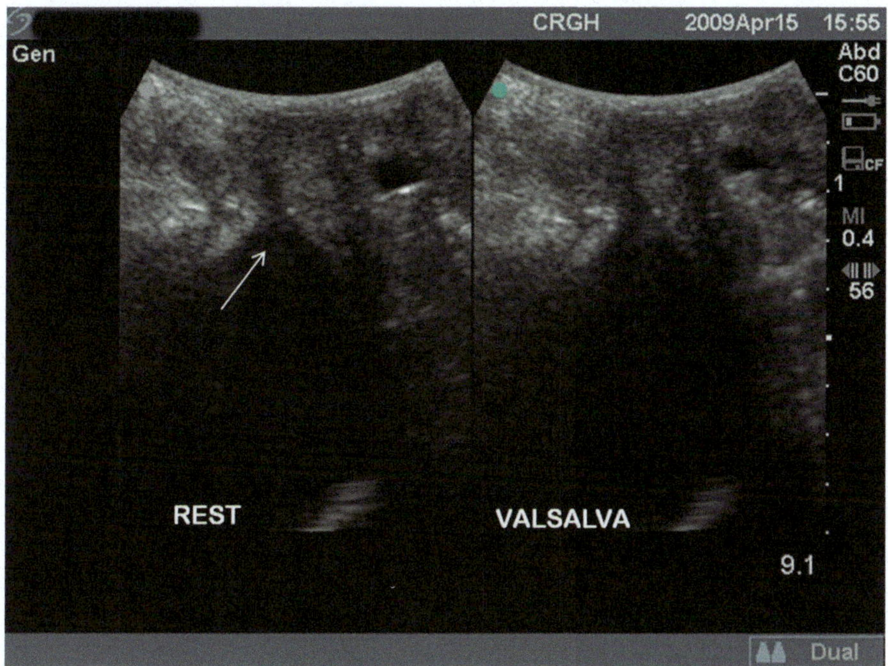

Fig. 5.8 Intrinsic urethral sphincter deficiency (ISD)- Transperineal ultrasound in a patient with severe urinary incontinence due to intrinsic urethral sphincter deficiency showing open bladder neck/proximal urethra at rest (*arrow*) and on Valsalva (*right image*). Note there is little urethral descent/mobility

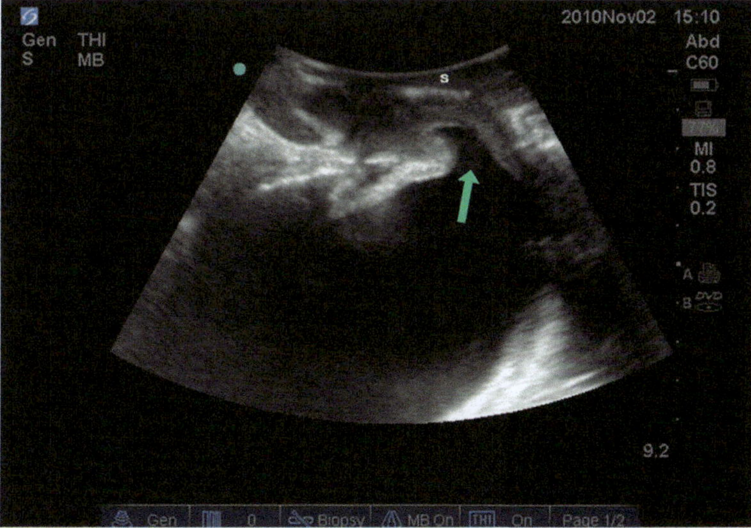

Fig. 5.9 Failed mid-urethral sling. Transperineal ultrasound in a patient with persisting urinary incontinence following mid-urethral sling surgery. Note open bladder neck/proximal urethra (*arrow*) due to intrinsic urethral sphincter deficiency (*s* sling)

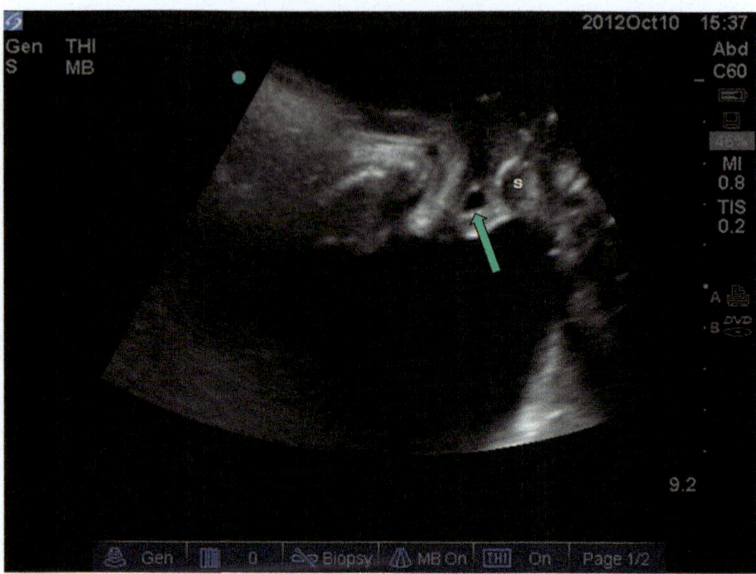

Fig. 5.10 Post injection of bulking agent. Transperineal ultrasound in the same patient (as Fig. 5.9) following injection of bulking agent (Bulkamid®, hypoechoic area- *arrow*) demonstrating coaptation of the proximal urethra above the level of the sling (*s*)

Comments The synthetic mid-urethral sling is the commonest surgical procedure worldwide for the treatment of stress urinary incontinence in women. However a proportion of patients will have suboptimal outcomes following sling surgery [1]. Possible causes of sling failure include technical reasons (sling misplacement), detrusor overactivity (either pre-existing, de-novo or secondary to obstruction) or the presence of significant urethral sphincteric deficiency (see Case 2).

Evaluation of the failed sling involves clinical examination and urodynamic assessment. Dynamic pelvic floor ultrasound has a role in evaluation of the position of the sling and urethral/bladder neck movement. The images (Fig. 5.9 and Video 5.6) illustrate an open bladder neck and proximal urethra consistent with the presence of urethral sphincter deficiency that is not corrected by the mid-urethral sling. This patient underwent injection of a bulking agent to the proximal urethra with successful coaptation of the urethra and improvement of her incontinence (Fig. 5.10 and Video 5.7).

Case 4: Recurrent Urinary Infections

A 43-year-old female presented with recurrent urinary infections following placement of a mid urethral sling 2 years previously for treatment of stress incontinence (Fig. 5.11a, b).

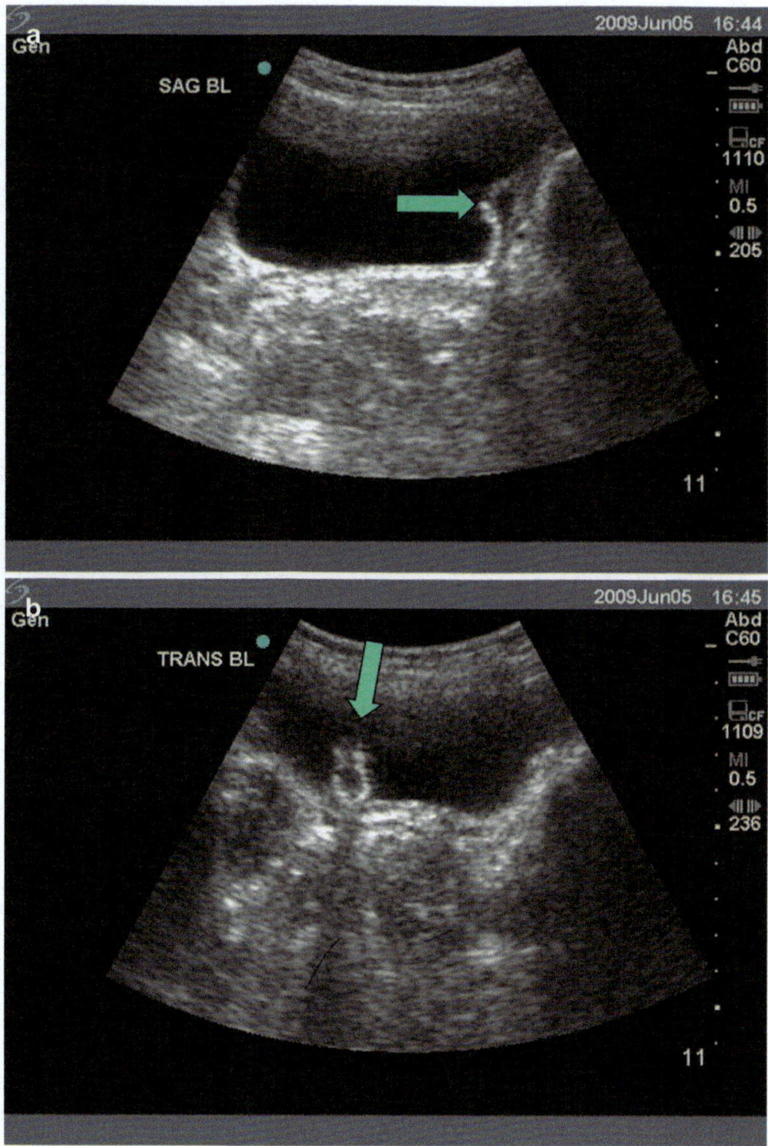

Fig. 5.11 (**a**, **b**) Transabdominal ultrasound of the bladder (sagittal and transverse images) demonstrating an eroded synthetic suburethral sling (*arrow*)

Comments In patients with urinary infections following placement of sling or mesh it is important to exclude erosion of mesh into the bladder or urethra, and also sling obstruction with incomplete bladder emptying. In this patient transabdominal ultrasound of the pelvis showed an eroded sling in the bladder (Fig. 5.11). This was confirmed on cystoscopy and the sling segment was removed endoscopically [2].

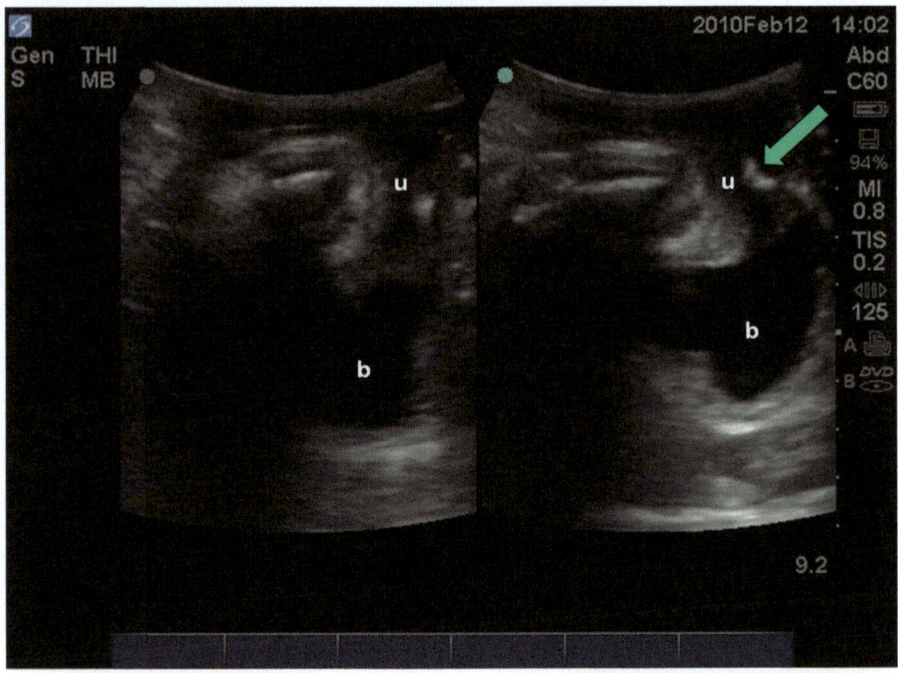

Fig. 5.12 Transperineal ultrasound images in a patient with voiding dysfunction post mid-urethral sling demonstrating angulation and kinking of the urethra by the sling (*right image- arrow*) during Valsalva (*b* bladder, *u* urethra)

Case 5: Voiding Dysfunction Post Sling Procedure

A 37-year-old female presented with symptoms of frequency, urgency, poor flow and incomplete bladder emptying following a retropubic mid-urethral sling procedure for stress incontinence. Transperineal ultrasound was performed to assess the sling's position (Fig. 5.12 and Video 5.8).

Comments The images demonstrate angulation and kinking of the urethra by the sling during straining/Valsalva. This is a common finding in obstructive slings. The patient subsequently underwent urethrolysis with the excision of a suburethral segment of the sling leading to resolution of her voiding dysfunction [3] (Video 5.9 confirms absence of the echogenic sling material behind the urethra following excision of a suburethral segment of sling).

Case 6: Neurogenic Bladder Dysfunction

A 45-year-old female with thoracic syringomyelia presented with urinary frequency, incontinence and recurrent urinary tract infections. These images (Fig. 5.13a, b) were obtained during a urodynamic study that demonstrated the presence of reduced detrusor compliance with a detrusor leak point pressure of 47 cm H2O.

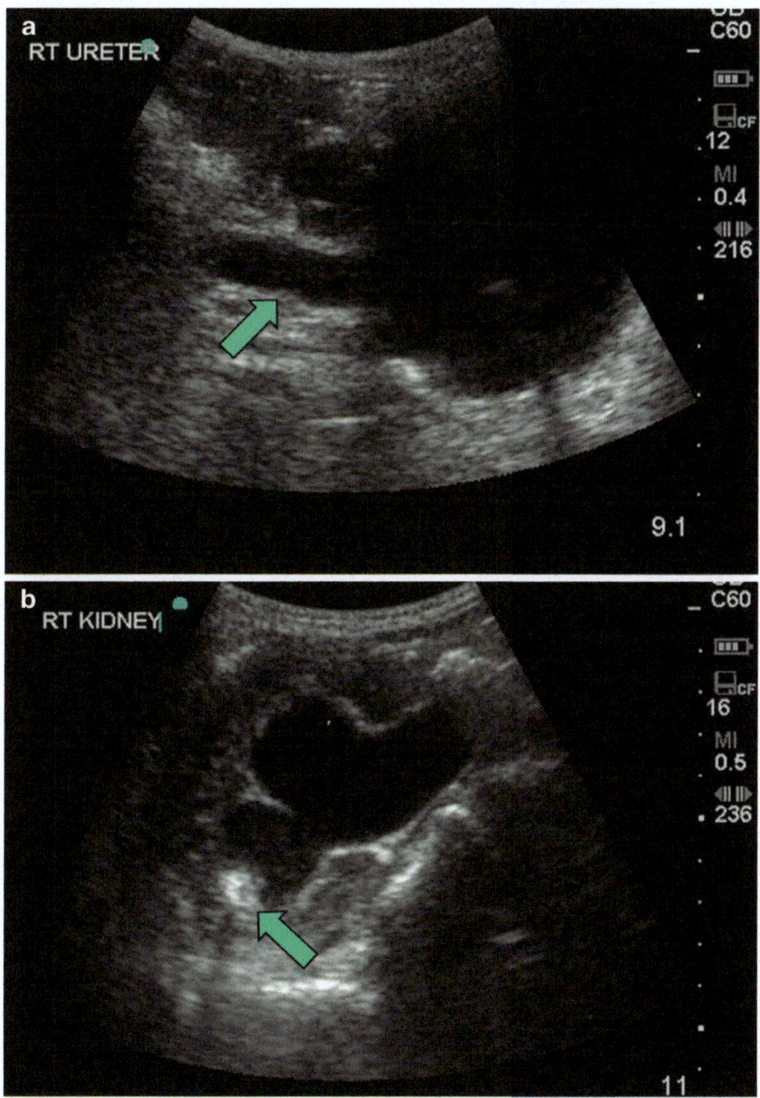

Fig. 5.13 (**a**, **b**) Neurogenic bladder. Transabdominal ultrasound images demonstrating trabeculated bladder (**a**) with dilated ureter (*arrow*) and hydronephrosis (**b**) with renal stone (*arrow*)

Comments Ultrasound is a good modality of imaging for video urodynamic studies. Apart from assessment of the bladder and urethra, it is easy to assess dilatation of the upper urinary tracts. In assessment of the neurogenic bladder, ultrasound has an advantage over fluoroscopy, as there is no need to transfer a patient with mobility impairment to a fluoroscopy table. However, it is generally not practical to image during the voiding phase. In this case of supra-sacral neurogenic bladder the imaging demonstrated the typical complications of high bladder storage pressures with a trabeculated bladder, vesico-ureteric reflux and renal stones.

References

1. Fong ED, Nitti VW. Mid-urethral synthetic slings for female stress urinary incontinence. BJU Int. 2010;106(5):596–608.
2. Chan LW, Tse VW. Unrecognised bladder perforation while placing a suburethral synthetic sling: a minimally invasive technique for removing an intravesical sling segment. BJU Int. 2005;95(1):187–8.
3. Tse V, Chan L. Outlet obstruction after sling surgery. BJU Int. 2011;108 Suppl 2:24–8.

Chapter 6
Practical Application of Ultrasound in the Assessment of Pelvic Organ Prolapse

Vincent Tse and Lewis Chan

Anatomy of Pelvic Organ Prolapse

Pelvic organ prolapse (POP) is a hernia of an adjacent pelvic viscus through attenuated supporting connective tissue into the vagina. Approximately one in nine women are reported to require POP surgery in their lifetime [1]. Risk factors include age, parity, prolonged second stage labour, connective tissue disorders and genetic factors such as defective collagen synthesis. A cystocele will result if the support of the anterior vaginal compartment is attenuated. A rectocele or enterorectocele will form if posterior vaginal compartment support is deficient. Apical weakness may lead to uterine prolapse, or an enterocele if the uterus is absent. Any combination of the above three areas can co-exist in any patient (Fig. 6.1). Transperineal ultrasound allows the clinician to visualize the three compartments of the pelvis in a simple and non-invasive fashion (see Chap. 5).

The Normal Female Pelvis

Figure 6.2 demonstrates the normal ultrasonic disposition of the female pelvic organs, namely, normal position of pubic symphysis, bladder, urethra, vagina, uterus, and rectum.

Electronic supplementary material The online version of this chapter (doi: 10.1007/978-3-319-04310-4_6) contains supplementary material, which is available to authorized users.

V. Tse, MBBS, MS, FRACS • L. Chan, MBBS(Hons), FRACS, DDU (✉)
Department of Urology, Concord Repatriation General Hospital, Sydney, NSW, Australia
e-mail: vincent.tse@sydney.edu.au; lewis.chan@sswahs.nsw.gov.au

L. Chan et al. (eds.), *Pelvic Floor Ultrasound: Principles, Applications and Case Studies*, DOI 10.1007/978-3-319-04310-4_6

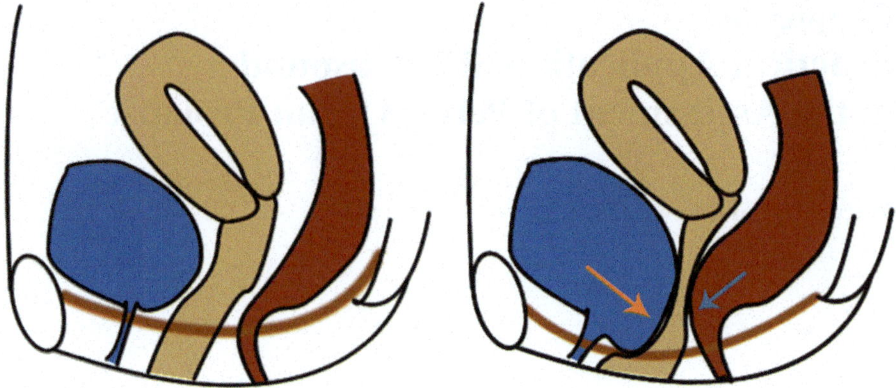

Fig. 6.1 Pelvic organ prolapse (POP). Weakness of the pelvic floor and supporting structures can result in POP (diagram on right) such as cystocele (*orange arrow*) and rectocele (*blue arrow*)

Practical Application of Ultrasound in Assessment of POP in Routine Clinical Practice

Although the use of pelvic ultrasound in assessing POP is not new and has been used in many academic centres in discovering and describing many anatomical defects utilizing many different research parameters [2–4], the pelvic floor reconstructive surgeon should also apply it in everyday clinical practice. One of the advantages of possessing ultrasound skills in routine clinical practice is that it can immediately add to the information which the clinician has already obtained in the history and physical examination. This advantage can come in the form of:

1. Assisting the clinician in confirming what is seen on physical examination;
2. More accurately delineating which organ(s) is prolapsed, especially in the posterior vaginal compartment when an enterocele component may not be immediately evident on physical examination;
3. Confirming and detecting the presence of any previous mesh repairs, as well as the current position and anchor points of the mesh, both in the static and dynamic situation. This may help in evaluation of mesh erosion into urethra, bladder or bowel.

Armed with this extra information immediately available at the bedside, the reconstructive surgeon can better understand the disease process behind each vaginal compartment, correlate it with the patient's symptomatology, and thus offer a more expedited and streamlined approach to management. In cases of recurrent POP after mesh repairs, ultrasound can often help the surgeon in understanding why the particular mesh failed, and this can allow the surgeon to reflect on whether it was a technical failure which he/she can improve on in future cases. This aspect has impact on quality improvement, continued professional development, and better patient care.

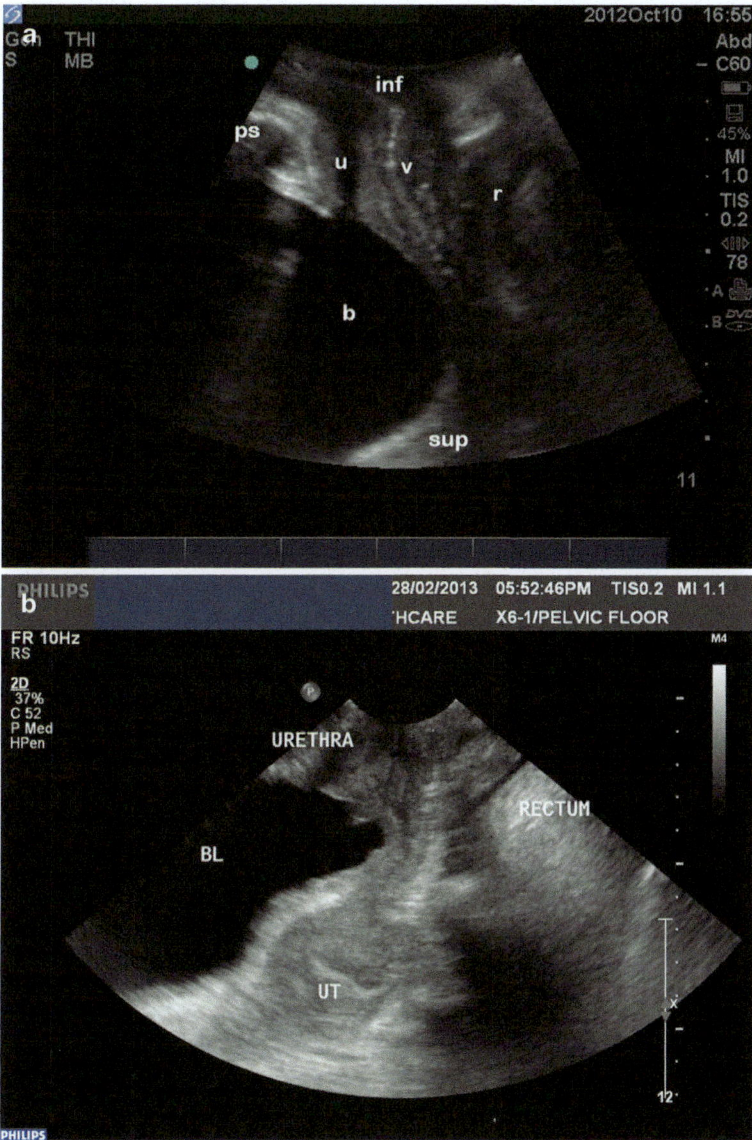

Fig. 6.2 (**a**, **b**) Sagittal transperineal ultrasound images demonstrating the three compartments of the pelvis. Bladder (*b*), urethra (*u*), vagina (*v*), rectum (*r*), pubic symphysis (*ps*), inferior/caudal (*inf*), superior/cranial (*sup*)

Technique of Transperineal Imaging of POP and Meshes (See Tips 6.1)

As for imaging mid-urethral slings, the transducer is placed on perineum, at the introitus (see Figs. 5.2 and 5.3). The bladder should be adequately filled. Valsalva manoeuvres are then used to assess the most dependent point of the prolapse in each of the three vaginal compartments so that a POP-Q assessment (Fig. 6.3) can be

Tips 6.1 Protocol and Tips for Transperineal Imaging of POP

- Lighting should be dim in the examination room
- Female chaperone should be present during the examination
- Imaging is often performed in the setting of urodynamic testing or in the office with at least 200 ml of bladder volume
- Static images obtained first of the disposition of the pelvic viscera
- Dynamic images with the patient performing a Valsalva maneuver are obtained, noting bladder neck/urethra mobility, presence of urodynamic stress incontinence or occult stress incontinence after reduction of the prolapse, also note the most dependent point of the prolapse for POP-Q assessment (see below diagram for POP-Q staging)
- Avoid excessive pressure on the introitus with the transducer during the examination as it may cause discomfort, and may obscures the severity of the prolapse
- Upper tract imaging (hydronephrosis/calculi) especially in higher stage prolapse or in a patient with unexplained deterioration in renal function
- Assessment of pelvic floor contraction
- Postvoid residual measurement if done in conjunction with urodynamics

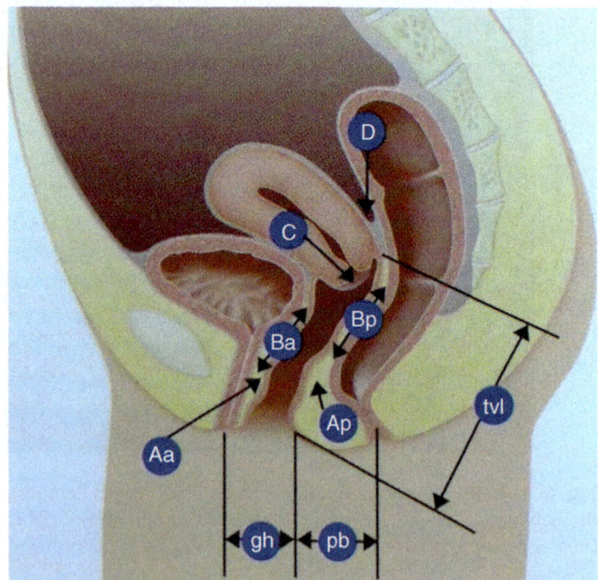

Fig. 6.3 POP-Q Quantification System (Image courtesy of American Medical Systems)

possible. Slings and pelvic organ prolapse meshes should be easily identified as a hyperechoic area in their respective areas (see Case 2). Scanning position should be in both supine and standing with full bladder if preferable, and take utmost care not to cause discomfort with pressure on the introitus which may also distort anatomy. Dynamic imaging will help to elicit location of the mesh, especially in failed cases, and to assess severity of the POP and how the mesh moves with straining.

1. Ordinate system (Fig. 6.3)	
Aa	Point on the anterior vaginal wall 3 cm from the hymen
Ba	The leading point on the anterior wall at maximal Valsalva with reference to the hymen
Ap	Point on the posterior vaginal wall 3 cm from the hymen
Bp	The leading point on the posterior wall at maximal Valsalva with reference to the hymen
C	Location of cervix or vaginal cuff with reference to the hymen
D	Location of posterior fornix or Pouch of Douglas with reference to the hymen
GH	Genital hiatus
PB	Perineal body
TVL	Total vaginal length

In the accompanying figure: the right side ordinates describe normal anatomical position of various points in a subject without prolapse, the left describe a patient with procidentia (i.e. total vaginal eversion)

2. Staging system	
Stage 0	No prolapse is demonstrated
Stage 1	The most distal portion of the prolapse is more than 1 cm above the level of the hymen
Stage 2	The most distal portion of the prolapse is 1 cm or less proximal or distal to the hymen
Stage 3	The most distal portion of the prolapse protrudes more than 1 cm below the hymen but protrudes no farther than 2 cm less than the total vaginal length (e.g. not all of the vagina has prolapsed)
Stage 4	Vaginal eversion is essentially complete

Advances in 3D/4D Pelvic Floor Ultrasound

In recent years, 3D ultrasound has introduced another dimension to ultrasound examination of the pelvis, and one can utilized this modality to allow more detailed examination of pelvic anatomy in relation to presence of mesh, especially its location in relation to urethra, bladder, rectum, and pubic symphysis (see Chap. 9).

The following cases illustrate the application of 2D transperineal pelvic floor ultrasound in the assessment of POP in routine clinical practice:

Case 1: 65 Year Old Lady Presenting with a Symptomatic Pop-Q Stage 3 Cystocele (Video 6.1, Fig. 6.4)

Comment This is a video clip of a transperineal ultrasound in the mid-sagittal plane, showing presentation of the cystocele from when the patient is at rest to when the patient achieves maximal Valsalva. At rest, the axis of the urethra is almost parallel to that of the vagina. The bladder is smooth in outline and there is no evidence of any intravesical lesions. There was no obvious POP evident at rest. However, as

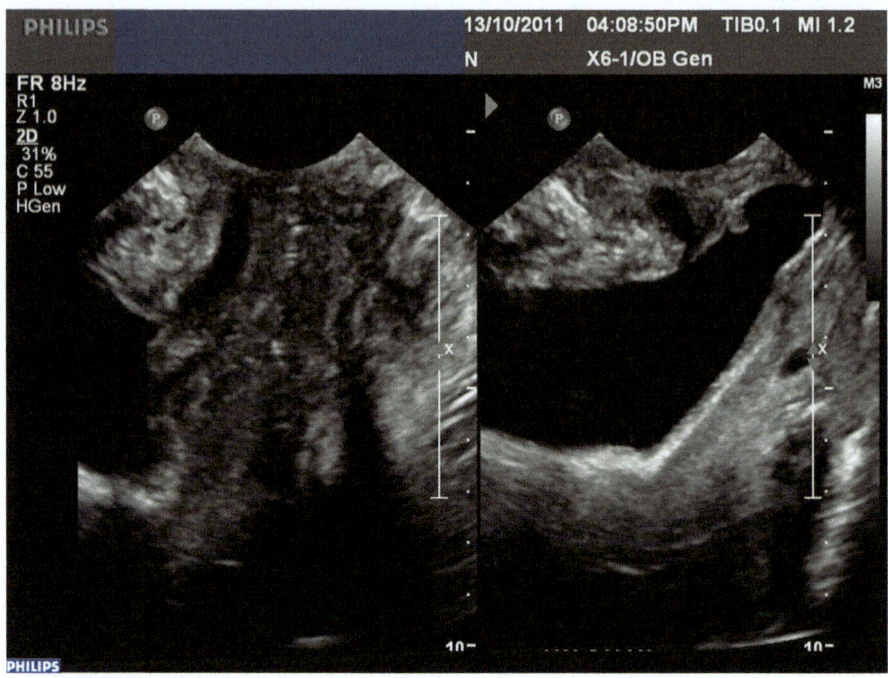

Fig. 6.4 Sagittal transperineal ultrasound images of POP-Q Stage 3 cystocele at rest (*left*) and at maximum Valsalva (*right*)

the patient starts to Valsalva, the urethral axis tilts caudally almost 90° during maximal Valsalva, and a large cystocele is seen protruding through the region of the introitus, reflecting poor lateral and central support of the bladder. The apical and posterior compartment remained relatively undisturbed during Valsalva.

Case 2: 72 Year Old Lady with Recurrent POP After a Previous Anterior Vaginal Mesh Repair and Mid-urethral Sling, Both via a Transobturator Approach (Video 6.2, Fig. 6.5)

Comment This case indicates further usefulness of having an ultrasound facility at the point of consultation to expedite diagnosis. At rest, this video clip showed a synthetic midurethral sling in situ, albeit located (or possibly migrated since it was placed) slightly more distal than the mid-urethra. The vagina is easily visible with its lumen. The mesh used in a previous transobturator cystocele repair can be seen as a curvilinear echogenicity adjacent to the bladder base. During Valsalva, (1) the mid-to-distal urethra showed dynamic compression against the sling to effect luminal coaptation; (2) the section of bladder that is adjacent to the mesh as well as the mesh

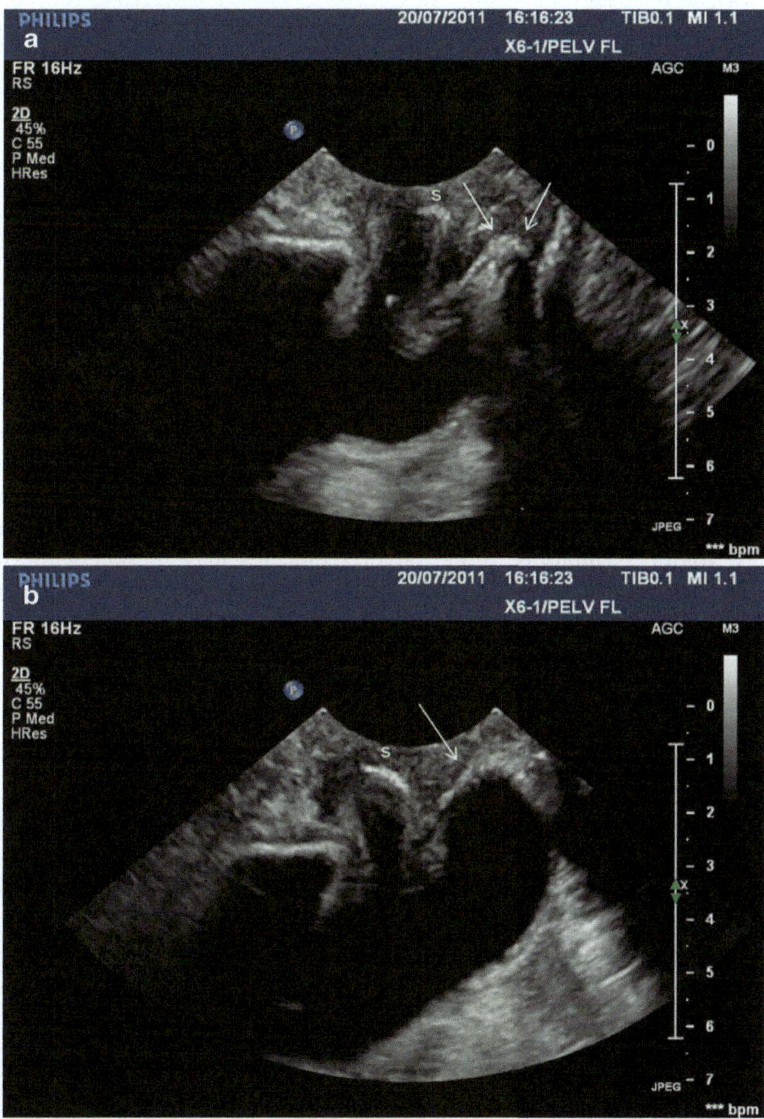

Fig. 6.5 Transperineal ultrasound images at rest (**a**) and on Valsalva (**b**) demonstrating recurrent POP post anterior vaginal mesh repair and mid urethral sling. Mid urethral sling (*s*), mesh (*white arrows*)

itself, can be seen to move together caudad at least 1.5–2.0 cm. This significant displacement of the mesh tells us that it is no longer attached to the lateral pelvic sidewall and has failed. The most dependent point of the prolapse had protruded past the mesh and presents as a large bulge beyond the introitus with straining. There is also associated descent of the vaginal apex, approximately 3 cm from its resting position during the Valsalva. One can see that the edict of "a picture is better than a thousand words" holds true in this instance whereby her continence as well as the reasons for her recurrent POP symptoms are clearly illustrated by a simple bedside ultrasound.

Case 3: Rectocele: 68 Year Old Lady with Bulge Symptoms as Well as Constipation and Sensation of Incomplete Evacuation (Videos 6.3 and 6.4, Fig. 6.6)

Comment This video clip (Video 6.3) demonstrate the presence of a Stage 2 (POP-Q) rectocele. Fecal material is echogenic and when the patient Valsalvas, one can see bulging of the posterior vaginal wall consistent with a rectocele. This is best demonstrated with the patient standing (also see Fig. 5.4) where the prolapse is seen to reach the introitus (Video 6.4) Note that this rectocele does not appear to have caused urethral compression during abdominal straining and this patient did not have any voiding symptoms. Some larger rectoceles may present with voiding symptoms due to urethral compression which will resolve after treating the rectocele. Note that an enterocele (Fig. 6.7) was not present during straining in this patient. Together with her history and physical examination, the images also show that underlying cause of her symptoms are unlikely to be due to rectal intussusception or mucosal prolapse, but most likely due to the rectocele.

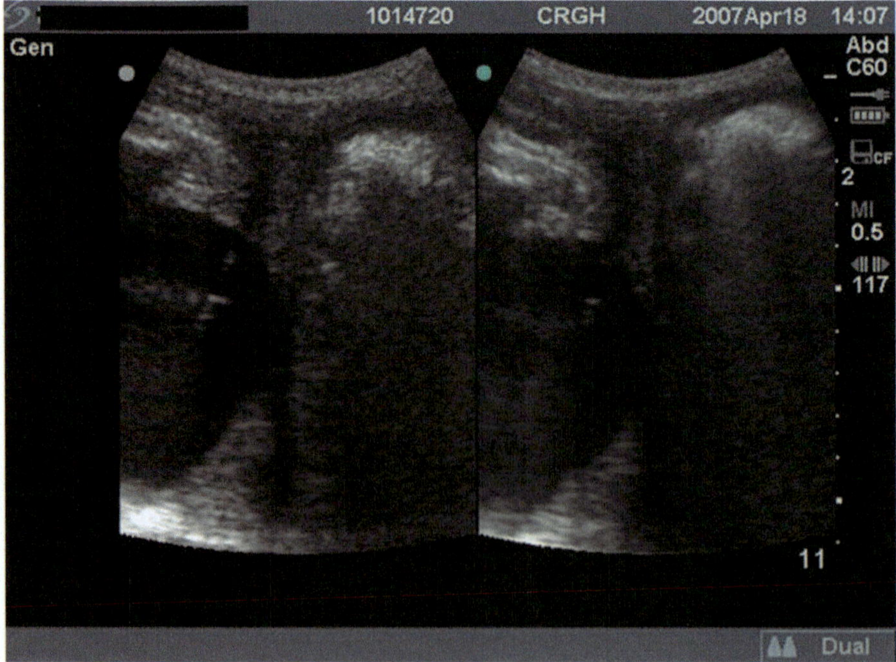

Fig. 6.6 Transperineal ultrasound images of rectocele at rest (*Left*) and on Valsalva (*right*)

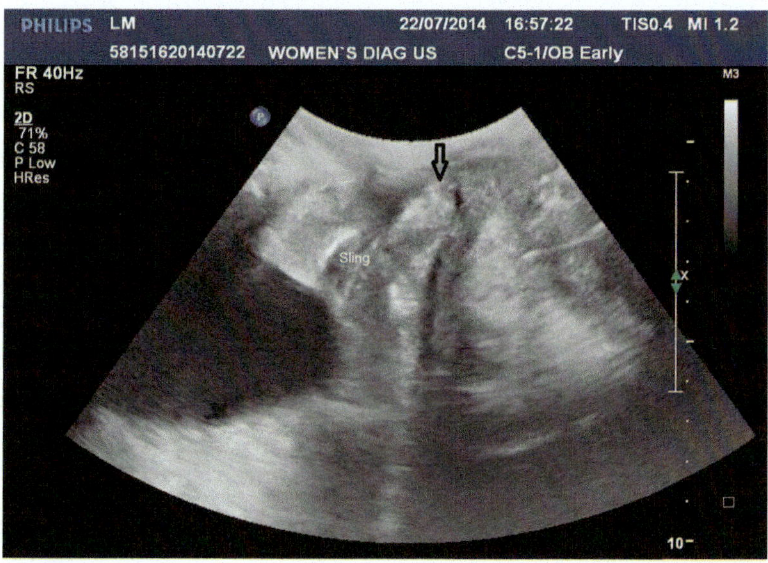

Fig. 6.7 Transperineal ultrasound image of an enterocele (*arrow*) presenting to the introitus in a patient with bulge symptoms. Note presence of mid-urethral sling

References

1. Olsen AL, Smith VJ, Bergstrom JO, et al. Epidemiology of surgically managed pelvic organ prolapse and urinary incontinence. Obstet Gynecol. 1997;89:501–6.
2. Weemholf M, et al. Effect of age on levator function and morphometry of levator hiatus in women with pelvic floor disorders. Int Urogynecol J. 2010;21(9):1137–42.
3. Constantinou C. Dynamics of female pelvic floor function using urodynamics, ultrasound and Magnetic Resonance Imaging (MRI). Eur J Obstet Gynecol Reprod Biol. 2009;144 Suppl 1:S159–65.
4. Huebner M, et al. Pelvic architectural distortions are due to pelvic organ prolapse. Int Urogynecol J Pelvic Floor Dysfunct. 2008;19(6):863–7.

Chapter 7
Ultrasound Imaging of Gynaecologic Organs

Stephanie The

Knowledge of the sonographic anatomy of female pelvic organs is important in the assessment of incontinence and the pelvic floor. A number of gynaecological conditions can present with stress or urge incontinence, and the presence of a large pelvic mass may worsen pelvic floor symptoms. This chapter outlines the technique of imaging of the female pelvic organs for the non-gynaecologist and common gynaecologic pathologies which may be encountered during pelvic ultrasound imaging.

The female pelvic organs can be imaged by transabdominal (Fig. 7.1) or transvaginal (Fig. 7.2) routes. Generally the best images are obtained by the transvaginal approach as the organs are closer to the intracavity transducer which is a high frequency transducer thus obtaining better quality images.

Technique of Transabdominal Imaging of the Pelvic Organs (Video 7.1)

Transabdominal ultrasound of the pelvic organs is generally performed with a full bladder. This allows for an overview of the entire pelvis (Fig. 7.1). A large pelvic mass may only be seen transabdominally and can be missed if only a transvaginal ultrasound is performed.

- Begin by scanning just above the pubic symphysis in the sagittal plane. Use the bladder as an acoustic window to the pelvis. Angle the transducer into the pelvis and identify the uterus (Fig. 7.3). Assess whether the uterus is anteverted or

Electronic supplementary material The online version of this chapter (doi: 10.1007/978-3-319-04310-4_7) contains supplementary material, which is available to authorized users.

S. The, MBBS, FRANZCOG, DDU, COGU
Department of Women's and Children's Health, Pelvic Floor Unit, Westmead Hospital, Sydney, NSW, Australia
e-mail: wdu@optusnet.com.au

L. Chan et al. (eds.), *Pelvic Floor Ultrasound: Principles, Applications and Case Studies*, DOI 10.1007/978-3-319-04310-4_7

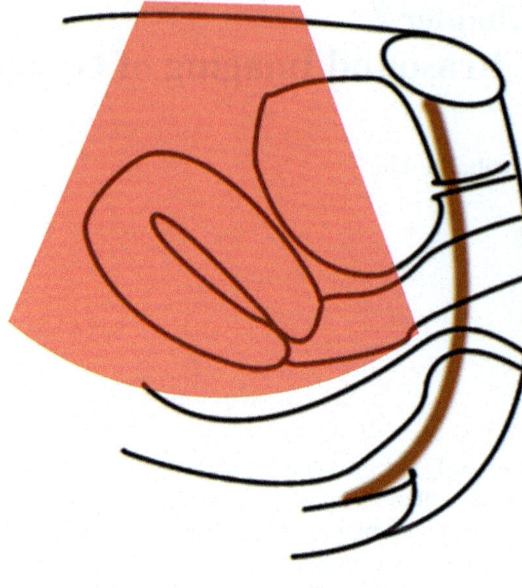

Fig 7.1 Transabdominal imaging of pelvic organs

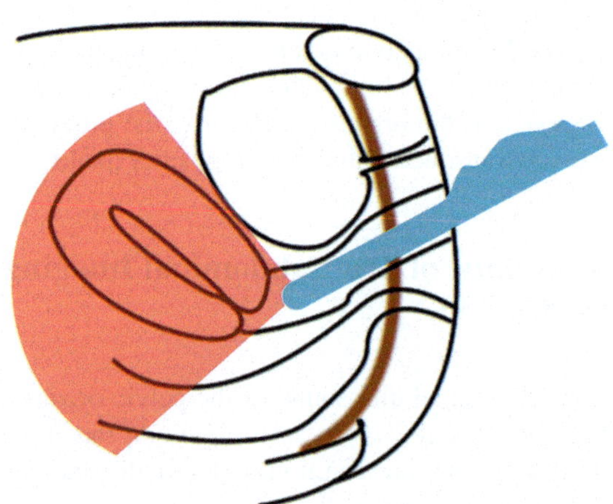

Fig 7.2 Transvaginal imaging of pelvic organs

retroverted. Look for any uterine masses by sweeping the transducer from one side to the other. Rotate the transducer 90° to assess the uterus in the transverse plane. Sweep the transducer up and down the uterus.

- The endometrium should be assessed in the sagittal plane from the endocervical canal to the fundus. Rotate the transducer and assess the endometrium in the transverse plane.
- Following assessment of the endometrium, angle the transducer laterally towards the adnexae to assess the ovaries. The ovaries are hypoechoic ovoid structures which are generally located between the uterus and the iliac vessels (Fig. 7.4). Examine the ovary in two planes and then assess the other ovary. Assess the adnexal regions and Pouch of Douglas.

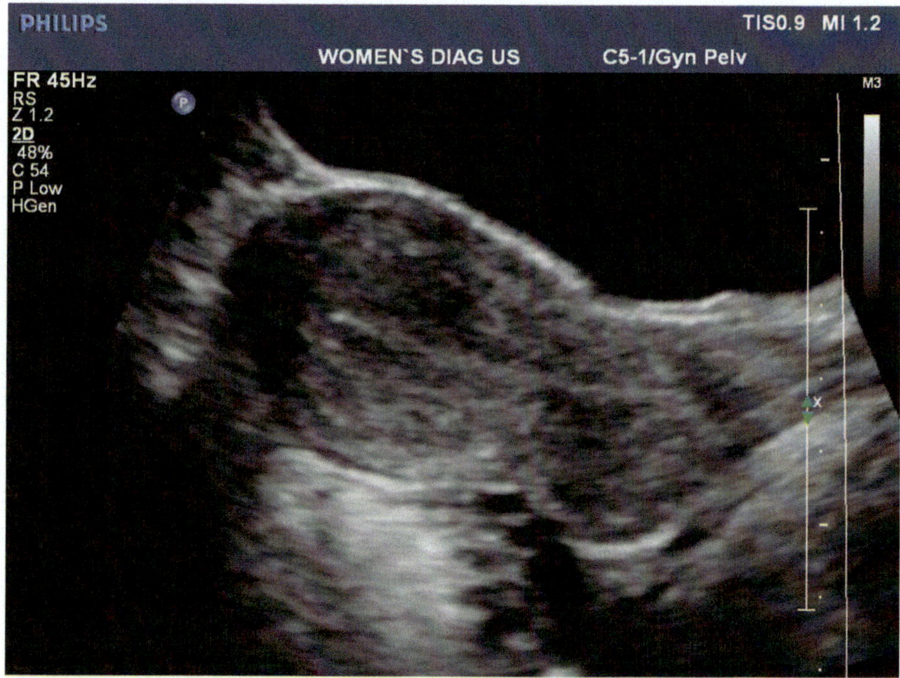

Fig 7.3 Transabdominal image of the uterus in the mid-sagittal plane

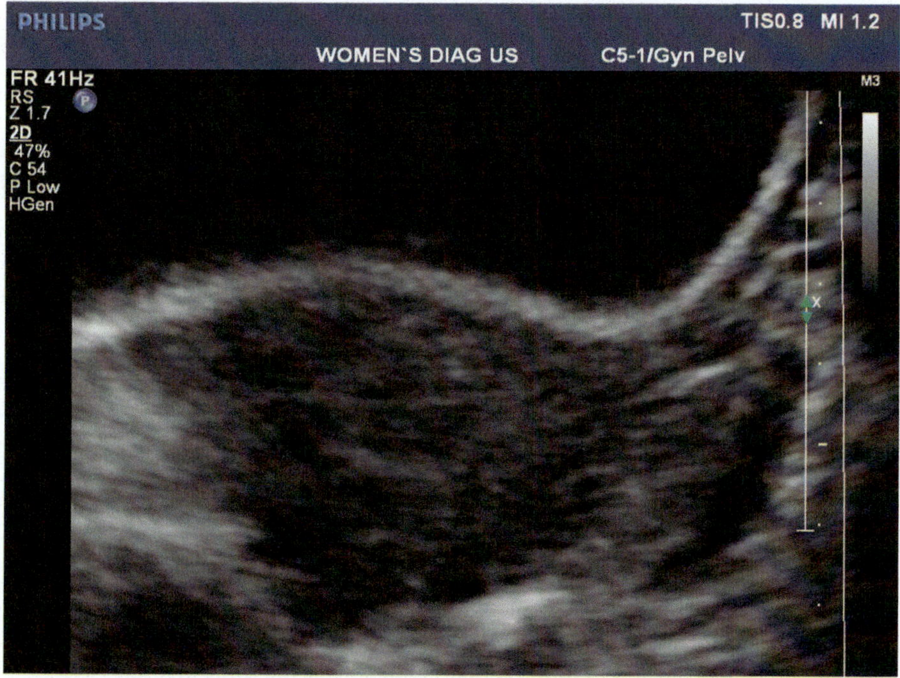

Fig 7.4 Transabdominal image of left adnexa showing the uterus and the left ovary

Transvaginal Assessment of Female Pelvic Organs (Video 7.2)

Transvaginal ultrasound scan is performed with an endocavity transducer. The patient should be asked to empty her bladder prior to the ultrasound scan.

- Begin by inserting the transducer in the sagittal plane to identify the uterus. To find the uterus, the transducer may need to be swept slightly to the left or right of the mid-sagittal plane or directed anteriorly or posteriorly.
- Once the uterus is identified, rotate the transducer so that a true mid-sagittal view of the uterus is obtained (Fig. 7.5). In the mid sagittal plane the endometrium should be seen from the cervix up to the fundus (calipers).
- Assess the uterus by sweeping from one side to the other in the sagittal plane and then cranially and caudally in the transverse plane to examine the whole uterus.
- The endometrium should be assessed in the sagittal plane from the endocervical canal to the fundus. Rotate the transducer and assess the endometrium in the transverse plane.
- Then look for the ovaries in the transverse plane by withdrawing the transducer out slightly and angling towards to the left or right fornix of the vagina. Sweep cranially and caudally to find the ovary. Assess the ovary in two planes then assess the other ovary.
- Look at the surrounding structures between the uterus and ovaries for any other adnexal masses.
- Return to the midline and angle the transducer posteriorly to assess for free fluid in the Pouch of Douglas.
- At the end of the examination, assess the vagina during withdrawal of the transducer from the vagina. Gartner's duct cysts are often only seen as the transducer is being removed.

The Normal Female Pelvis

In order to recognize pelvic pathology, it is important to be familiar with the anatomy of the normal pelvis. The following are images of the normal pelvis.

Figure 7.5 shows an anteverted uterus, where the fundus of the uterus is directed towards the bladder. The majority of women have an anteverted uterus. In this image the endometrial stripe is seen in the proliferative phase (first half of the menstrual cycle) as a triple layer appearance. The uterus is usually 6–10 cm in length when measured from the cervix to the fundus in a menstruating woman. There is a Nabothian follicle in the cervix (blue arrow). These are commonly seen and is a normal finding.

Figure 7.6 shows a retroverted uterus, where the fundus of the uterus is directed away from the bladder. In this image the uterus is in the secretory phase of the menstrual cycle. The endometrium has lost the triple layer appearance and is thick and echogenic (blue arrow).

Figure 7.7 is of an anteverted uterus in the menstrual phase of the cycle. The endometrial echo is seen as a thin, regular echogenic stripe (blue arrow).

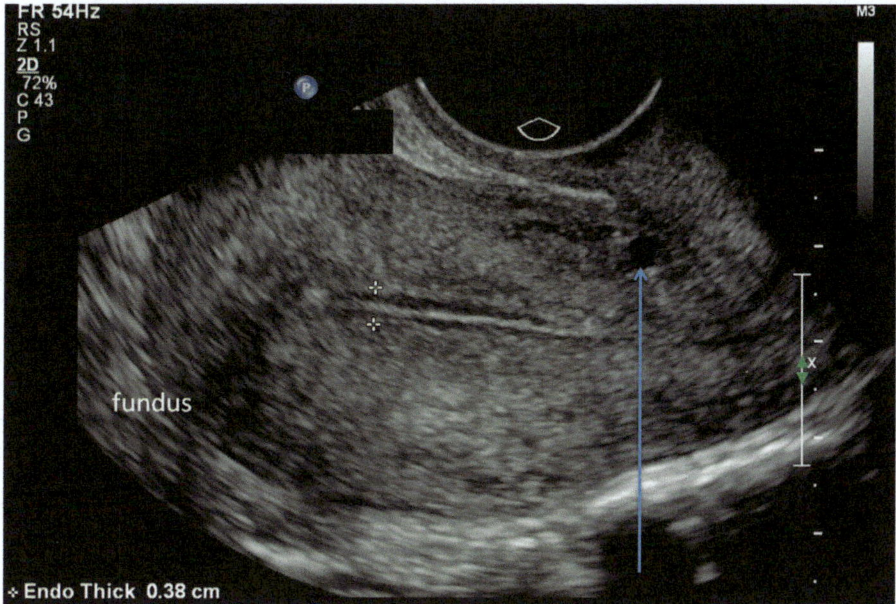

Fig. 7.5 Transvaginal image of an anteverted normal uterus in the mid sagittal plane

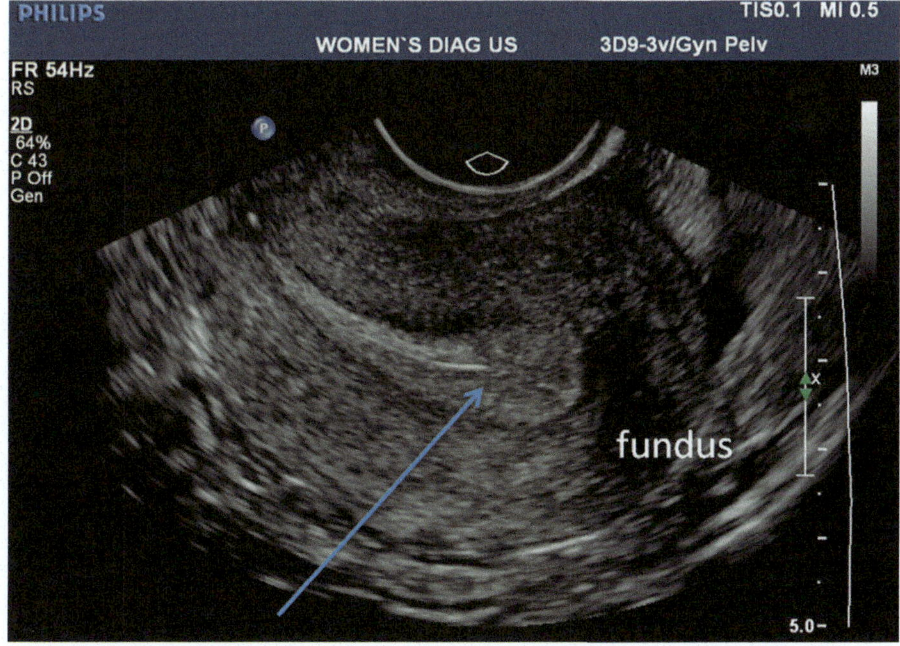

Fig 7.6 Transvaginal image of a retroverted normal uterus in the mid sagittal plane

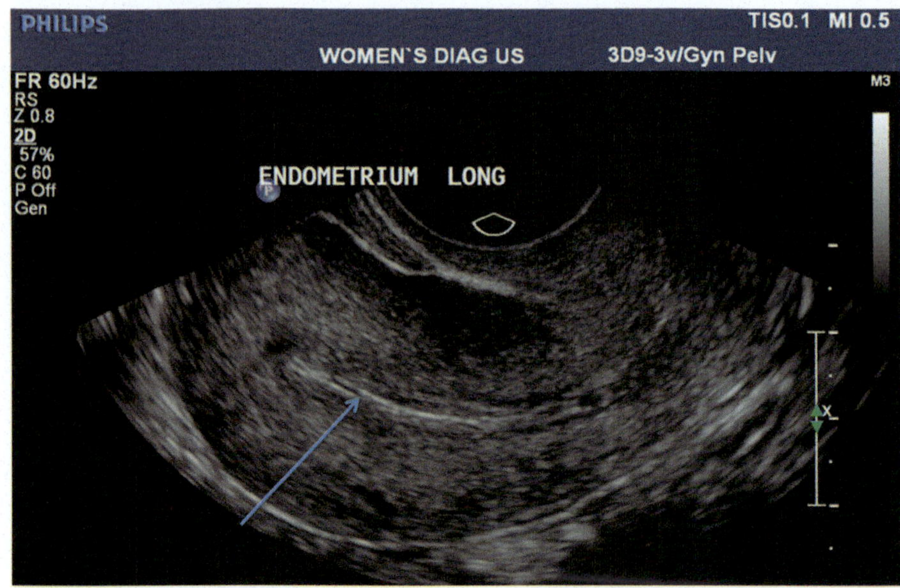

Fig. 7.7 Transvaginal image of a normal uterus in the menstrual phase of the cycle

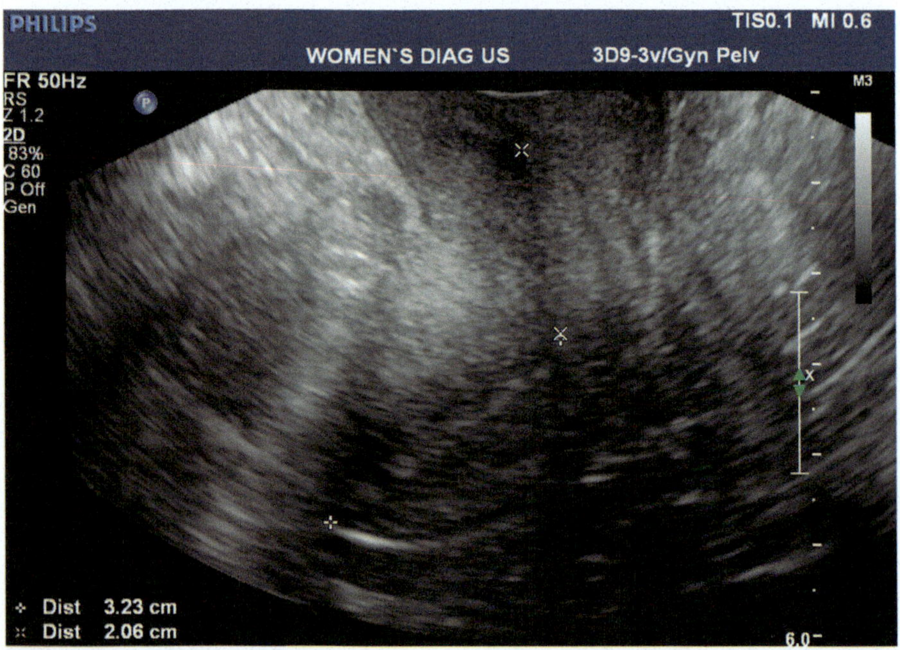

Fig. 7.8 Transvaginal image of a normal postmenopausal uterus

The postmenopausal uterus is small and should be 4–6 cm in length, with a thin endometrial stripe. The endometrium should measure <4 mm in thickness (Fig. 7.8).

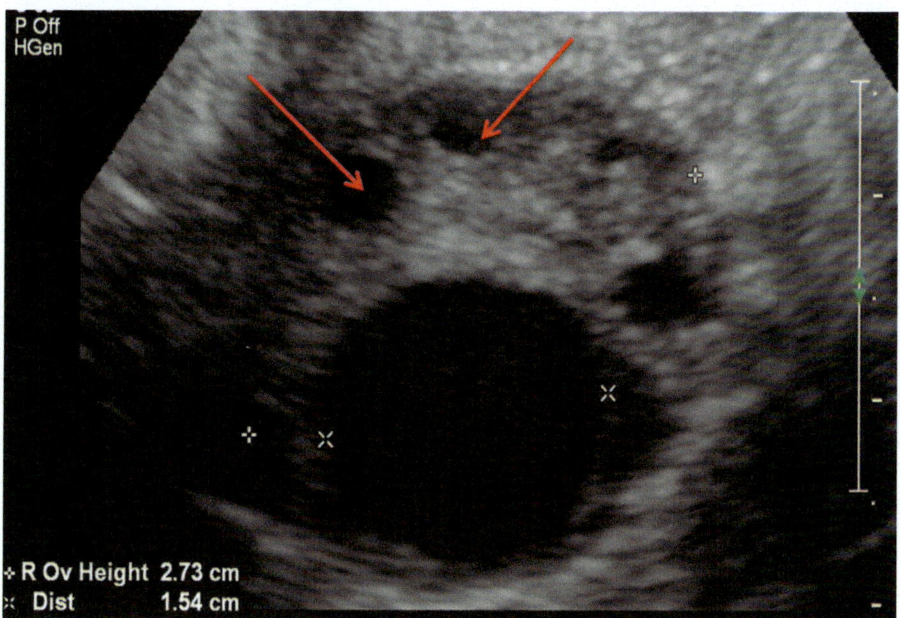

Fig. 7.9 Transvaginal image of a normal ovary in a woman of reproductive age

In this image of a normal ovary (Fig. 7.9) it can be seen as an oval hypoechoic structure. A few follicles can be identified – red arrows (usually about 6). There is a dominant follicle which measures 15.4 mm in diameter (calipers).

The normal ovary is usually about 4 × 3 × 2 cm in size in a woman of reproductive age. The ovary is usually found lateral to the uterus on each side, lying between the uterus and the iliac vessels. Occasionally the ovary is in the Pouch of Douglas or superior to the uterus.

Figure 7.10 is an image from a postmenopausal woman where the ovary is small and has little or no follicular activity.

Notes:

The uterus may be anteverted or retroverted. However the majority of women have an anteverted uterus.

The endometrium should be able to be visualised from the endocervical canal to the fundus of the uterus.

Common Pelvic Pathology

The following conditions are not meant to be an exhaustive list of pathology that may be encountered in the pelvis, but rather a short list of the more common pathologies that may be encountered in pelvic imaging. The general principles for managing some of the commonly encountered pathologies for the non-gynaecologist are outlined in Tips 7.1.

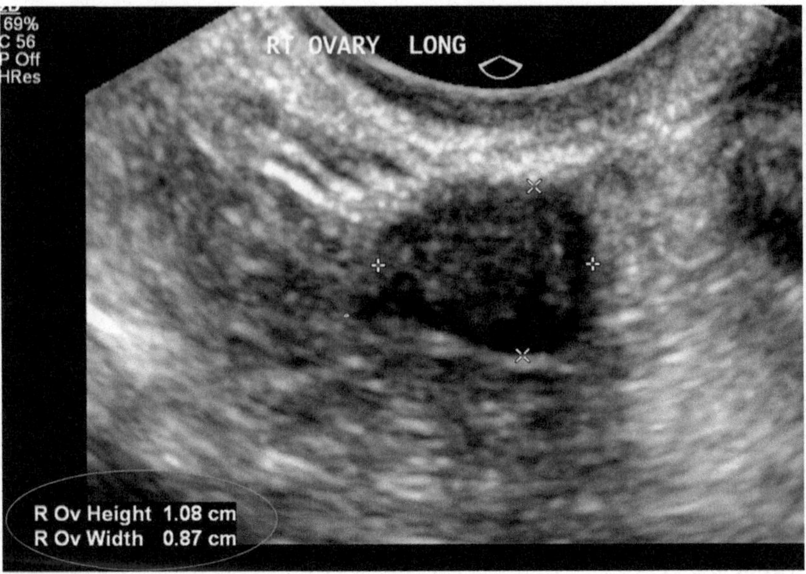

Fig. 7.10 Transvaginal image of a normal postmenopausal ovary

Tips 7.1 Keypoints in Imaging of Gynaecologic Organs for Non-gynaecologists

- Use the bladder and uterus as a guide to orientation in the pelvis (the bladder is anterior and the rectum posterior).
- Fibroids are common – they only need removal if the patient is symptomatic because of heavy bleeding (menorraghia) or has pressure symptoms, such as prolapse or incontinence.
- The endometrium should be <4 mm thick in a postmenopausal woman. Gynaecologic referral should be considered if endometrial thickness is >4 mm or the woman has postmenopausal bleeding
- Simple cysts <5 cm – usually functional and will resolve
- All other cysts need referral unless the appearance suggest a haemorrhagic corpus luteum (Fig. 7.19).

Leiomyomas (Fibroids)

These are common benign tumours arising from the smooth muscle cells of the uterus. Even though they are seen in up to 50 % of women, they are mostly asymptomatic. However fibroids can cause symptoms such as menorrhagia or pressure symptoms such as urinary frequency (especially if large).

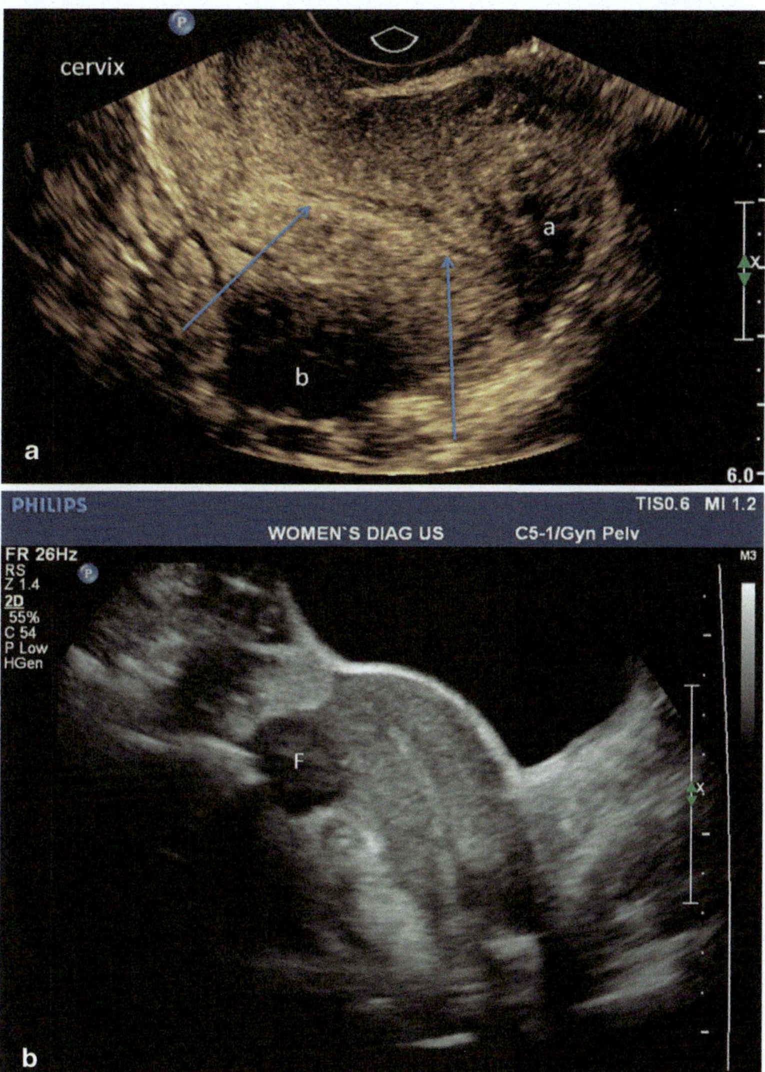

Fig. 7.11 (**a**) Transvaginal image of a uterus which contains an intramural fibroid (**a**) and a subserous fibroid. (**b**) Transabdominal image of an anteverted uterus with a posterior subserous fibroid (*F*)

Sonographically, fibroids are hypoechoic masses and can be intramural (within the walls of the uterus), subserosal (located under the serosal surface and distorting the serosal surface) or submucous (the fibroid projects partially or completely into the uterine cavity).

Figure 7.11a shows a retroverted uterus with an intramural fibroid (a) in the posterior myometrium. Here the fibroid is intramural because it is located wholly

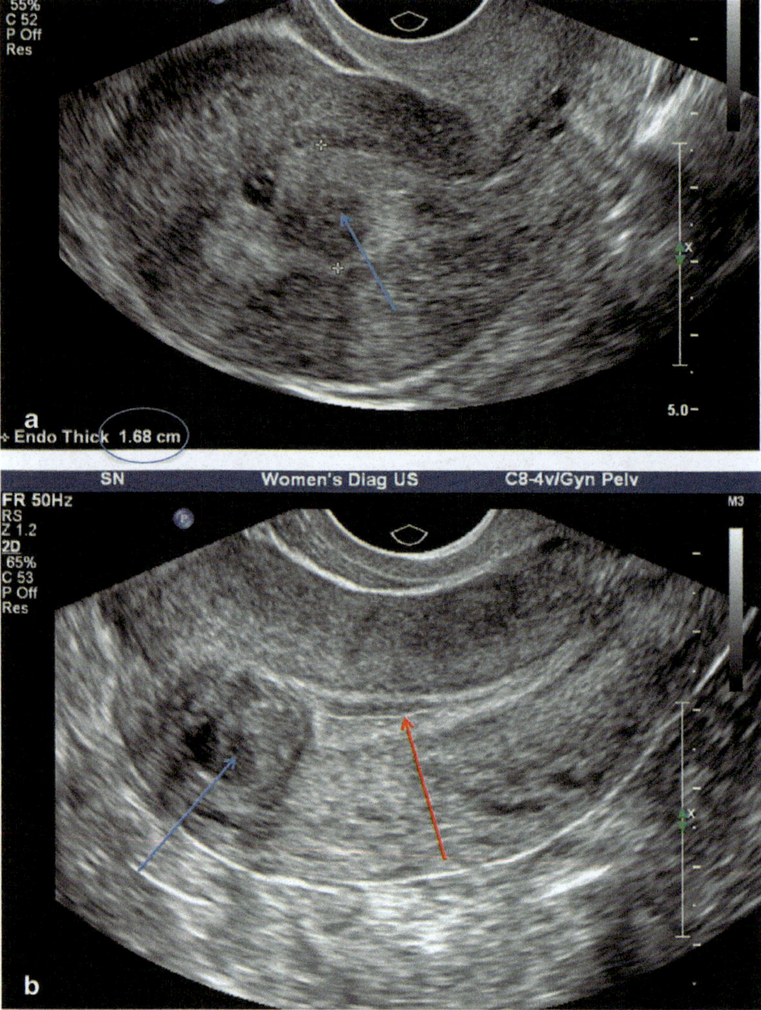

Fig 7.12 (**a**, **b**) Submucous fibroids

within the walls of the uterus. There is also a subserous fibroid (b) which distorts the anterior serosal surface. The fibroids can be seen as well defined hypoechoic solid masses with posterior shadowing. The blue arrows are pointing to the endometrium.

Figure 7.12a shows a thickened endometrium that measures 16.8 mm. This is due to the presence of a well defined hypoechoic mass within the endometrium (blue arrow), which is a small fibroid. As the fibroid is within the endometrial cavity it is classified as a submucous fibroid. Figure 7.12b shows a submucous fibroid (blue arrow) disrupting the endometrium (red arrow).

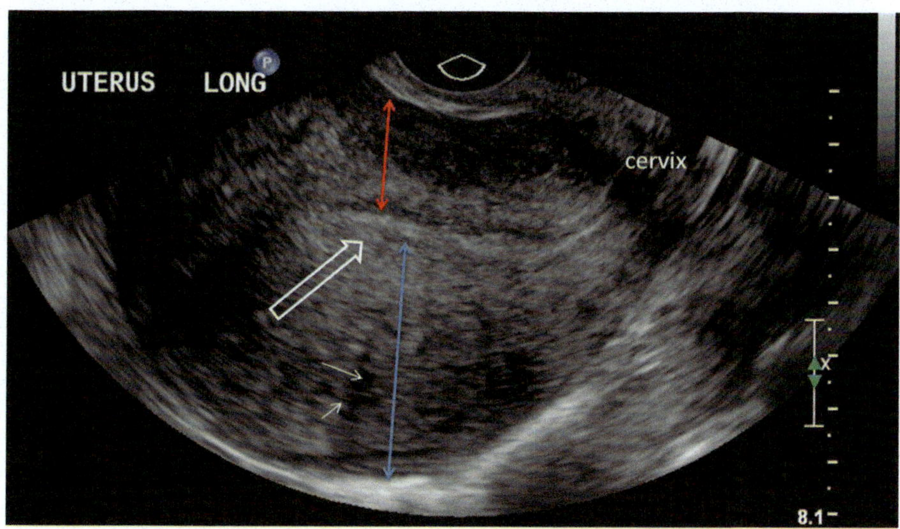

Fig. 7.13 Transvaginal image of a uterus with adenomyosis

Adenomyosis

This condition arises as a result of ectopic endometrial tissue within the myometrium. The benign invasion of the myometrium can result in smooth muscle hyperplasia. Women with adenomyosis may complain of menorrhagia or dysmenorrhea.

Figure 7.13 shows a bulky uterus with a thick posterior uterine wall. Compare the thickness of anterior wall (red arrow) to the posterior wall (blue arrow). Here the myometrium has a coarse heterogenous echotexture with some tiny myometrial cysts (white arrows) and streaky acoustic shadowing. The endometrium and its junction with the myometrium is often poorly defined (large arrow).

Intrauterine Contraceptive Device (IUCD)

Figure 7.14 shows an IUCD which is visualized as a linear echogenic structure within the endometrial cavity (red arrow) with shadowing posteriorly (blue arrow).

Endometrial Polyp

These occur as a localized overgrowth of the endometrium and are seen as a protrusion into the endometrial cavity. Polyps can also arise as a result of tamoxifen treatment. Endometrial polyps are generally benign, but can cause abnormal bleeding such as intermenstrual bleeding, metorrhagia and infertility.

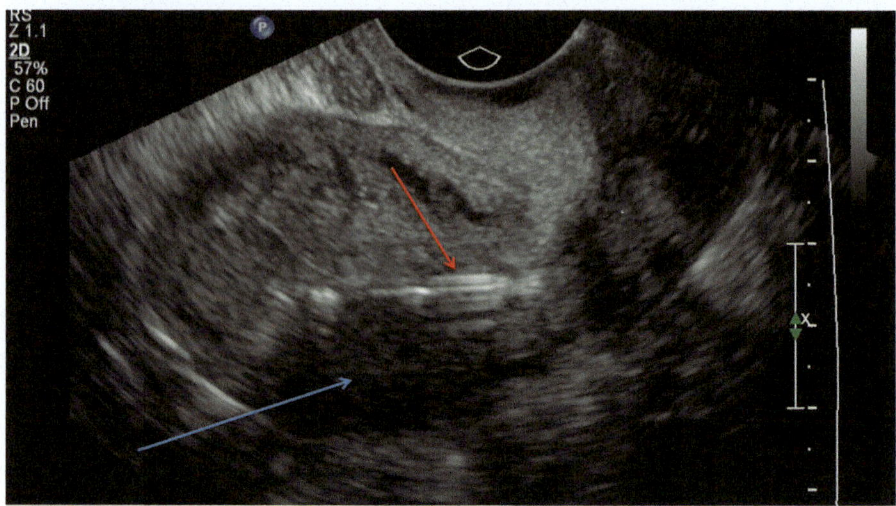

Fig. 7.14 Image of a uterus which contains and intrauterine contraceptive device

Polyps are best seen in the early proliferative phase of the cycle, when the endometrium is the thinnest and most hypoechoic.

In Fig. 7.15a an endometrial polyp can be seen as a small round echogenic mass within the endometrium (blue arrow). Application of Power Doppler shows the presence of a small feeding vessel within the mass.

The presence of the polyp (blue arrow) is confirmed with infusion of saline into the cavity (Fig. 7.15b).

Endometrial Hyperplasia

Endometrial hyperplasia is a thickening of the endometrium which is caused by hyperplasia of the endometrial glands.

In Fig. 7.16, the endometrium is unusually thick and echogenic (blue arrow) with some cystic spaces (red arrows).

Endometrial Carcinoma

In this postmenopausal woman (Fig. 7.17) who presented with vaginal bleeding, the endometrium is thickened (blue arrow) and there is invasion to the serosal surface of the uterus (red arrow).

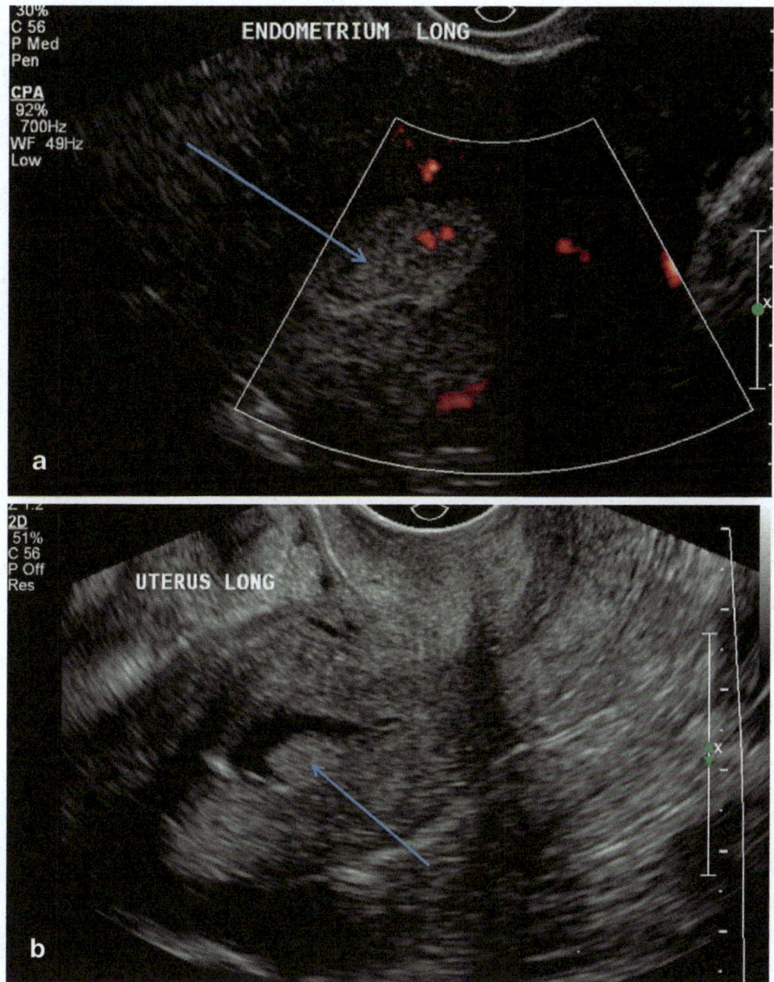

Fig. 7.15 (**a**) Transvaginal ultrasound of a uterus which contains an endometrial polyp (*blue arrow*). (**b**) Saline sonohysterogram demonstrating the endometrial polyp

Ovarian Cysts

Simple Ovarian Cyst

This image (Fig. 7.18) shows a thin walled cyst which is filled with anechoic fluid. The diameter of the cyst is 42.7 mm, which is >25 mm. Up to 25 mm, these anechoic structures may be a follicle. There is a crescent of normal ovarian tissue seen (arrow).

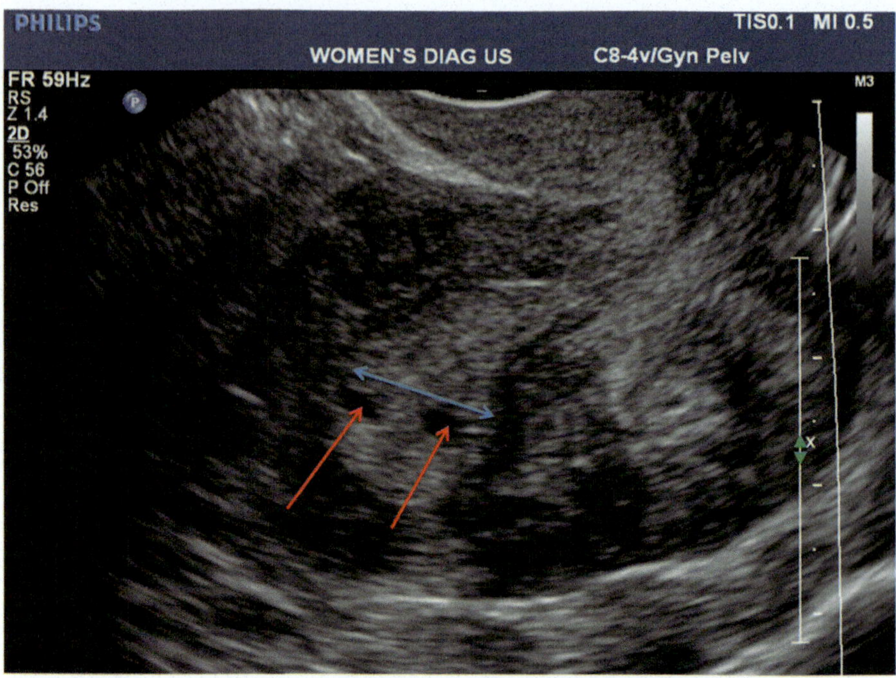

Fig. 7.16 Transvaginal ultrasound image of a uterus which has endometrial hyperplasia

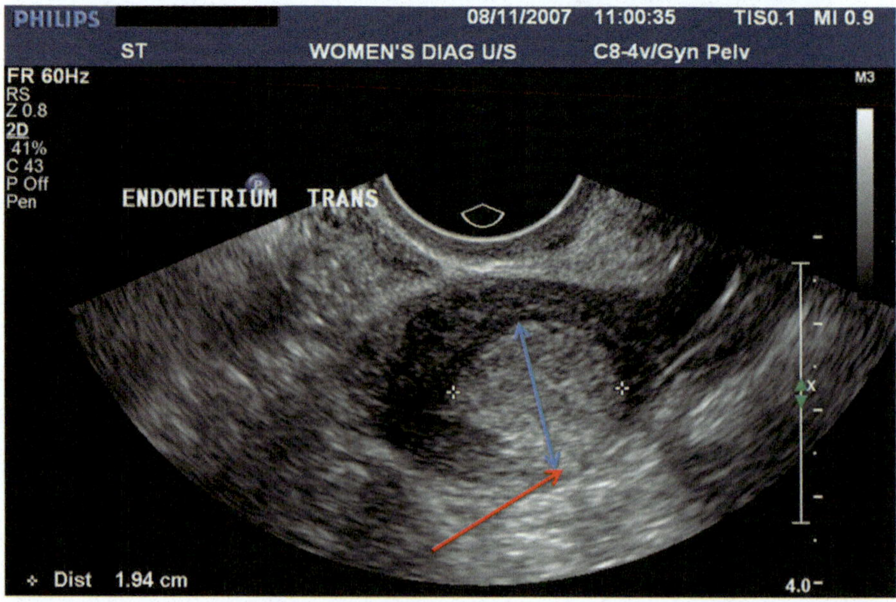

Fig. 7.17 Transvaginal image of a postmenopausal uterus in the transverse plane with an endometrial carcinoma

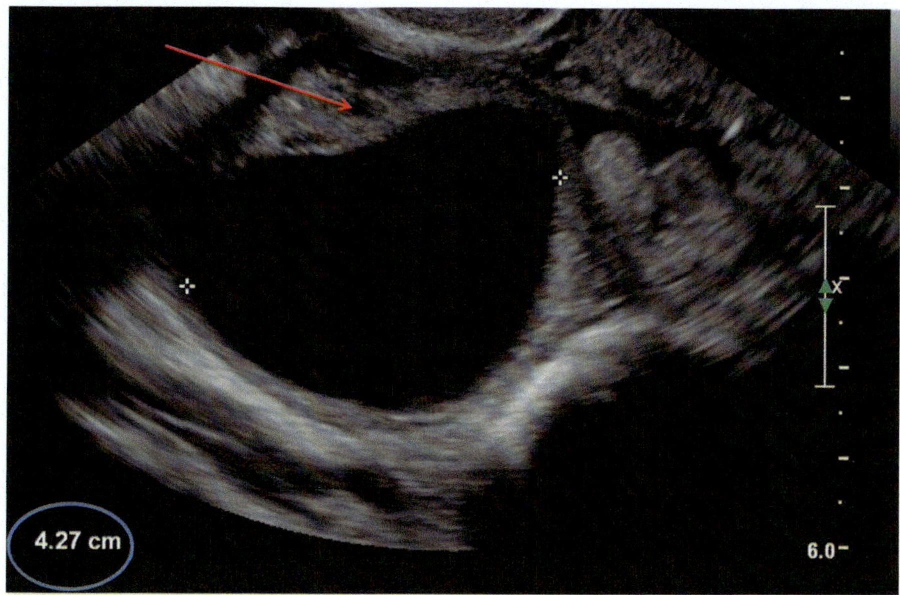

Fig. 7.18 Simple ovarian cyst

Ovarian cysts are often functional (especially if they are <5 cm) and usually resolve with time. Cysts are only classified as simple if they contain fluid which is completely anechoic, and do not contain septations, solid elements or nodules (see Tips 7.2).

Tips 7.2 Sonographic Criteria for Simple Cysts (Also See Chap. 1)

- Thin, smooth wall
- Anechoic contents
- No septa or nodules
- Posterior acoustic enhancement

Haemorrhagic Cysts (Corpus Luteal Cyst) arise after ovulation and are therefore most commonly seen in the second half of the menstrual cycle.

Figure 7.19 is an image of a haemorrhagic cyst with a typical heterogenous 'lacy' appearance with thin walls. Colour Doppler imaging shows circumferential peripheral vascularity ("ring of fire").

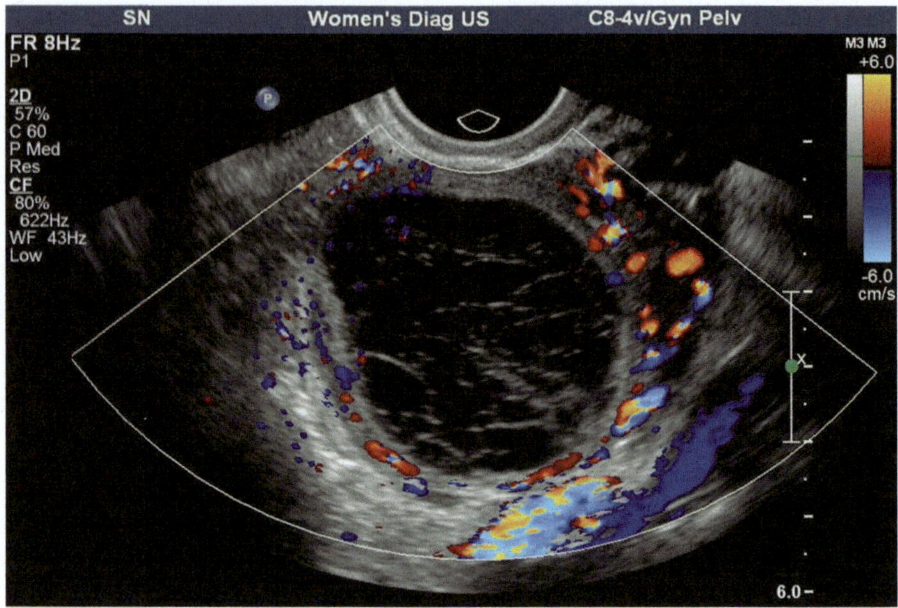

Fig. 7.19 Corpus luteal cyst

Polycystic Ovaries

The Rotterdam Consensus Statement defines the polycystic ovary as having 12 or more follicles measuring between 2 and 9 mm in diameter, and/or an ovarian volume of greater than or equal to 10 cc [1].

Figure 7.20 shows an ovary with multiple follicles (blue arrows) which are peripherally arranged in the ovary. The stroma is echogenic (red arrow), which is also often seen in a polycystic ovary.

Endometriomas

Endometriosis occurs as a result of the presence of functioning endometrial tissue outside the uterus. This can result in a cystic structure, known as an endometrioma.

Figure 7.21 is an ovary containing a well defined cystic mass which is filled with homogenous echogenic material with a characteristic "ground glass" appearance (red arrow). This cyst has well defined walls, as well as a fluid – fluid level (blue arrow).

Mature cystic teratomas (Dermoid) arise from the germ cell elements of the ovary. They are mostly derived from ectodermal components and therefore often

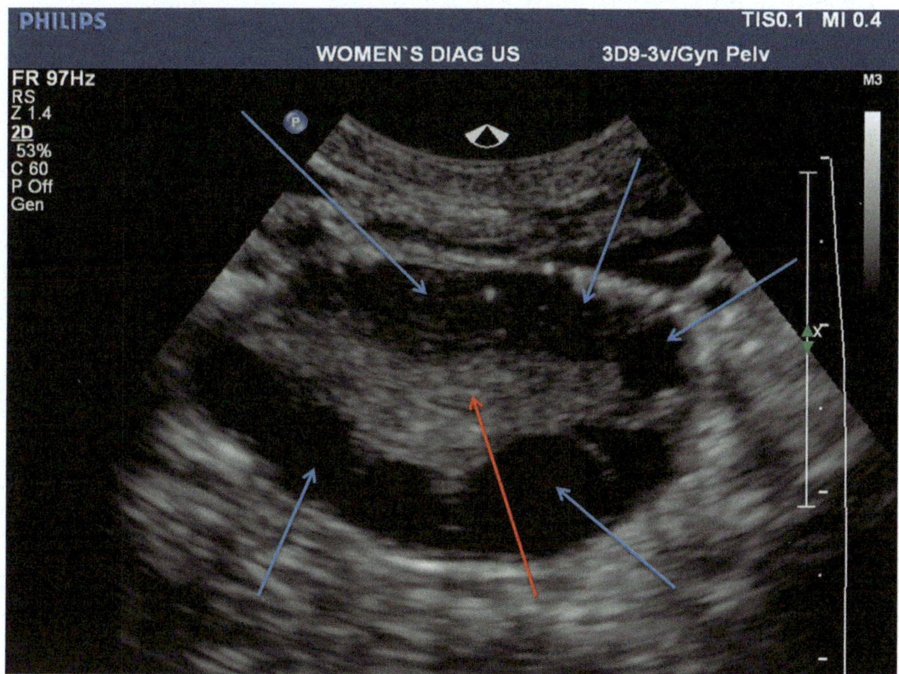

Fig 7.20 Transvaginal ultrasound image of a polycystic ovary

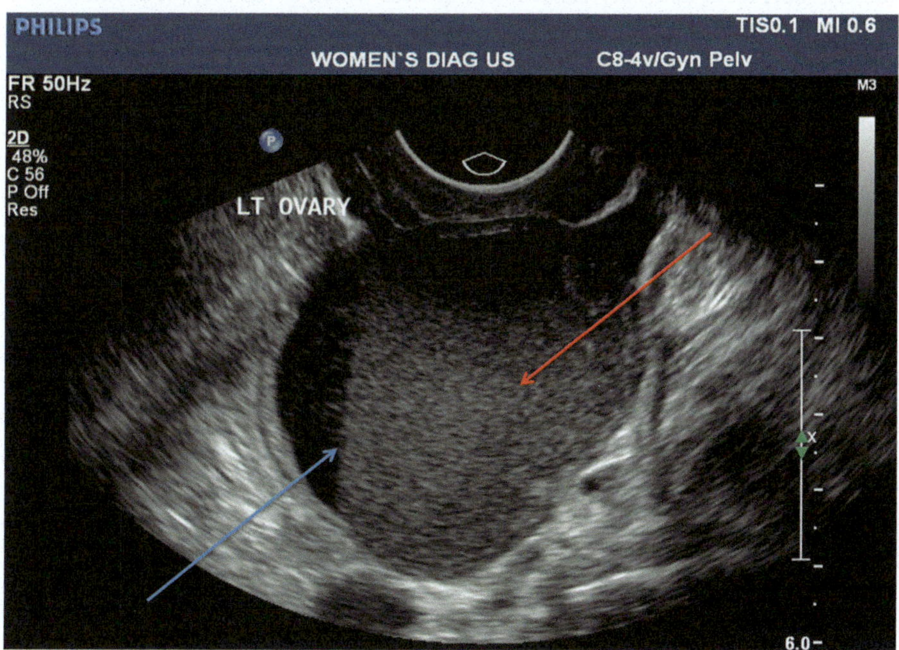

Fig. 7.21 Transvaginal image of an ovary which contains an endometrioma

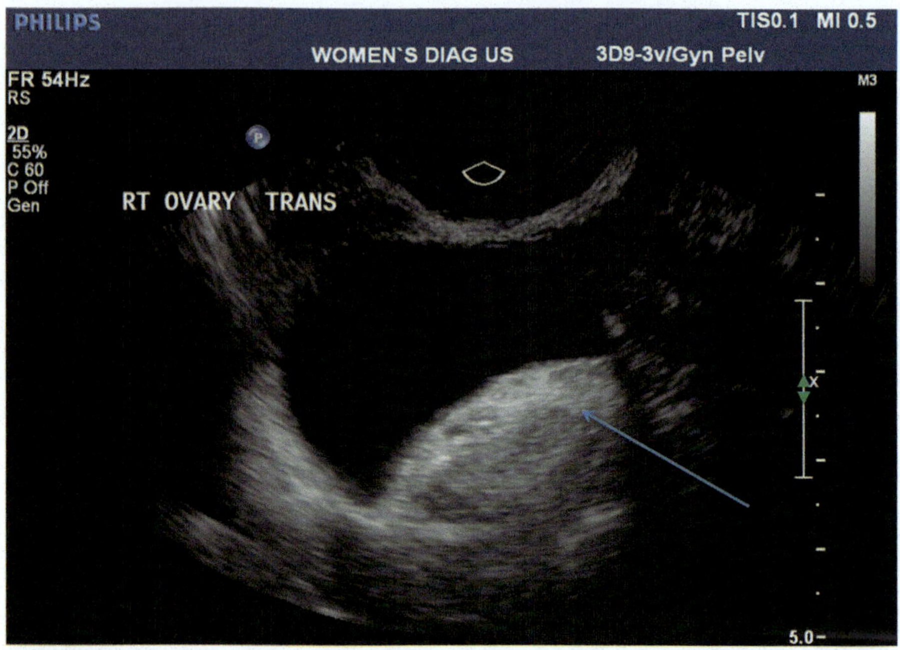

Fig. 7.22 Transvaginal image of an ovary which contains a dermoid cyst

contain hair, teeth and fatty sebaceous material which gives them a characteristic ultrasound appearance.

Figure 7.22 shows some of the features typically seen with a dermoid. These tumours are usually mostly cystic with mixed solid and cystic components. Typical features can include a highly echogenic mass (arrow) with posterior acoustic attenuation due to the fatty component of sebaceous material in the cyst. There is a fluid-fluid level.

Another feature (not shown) include multiple thin echogenic lines caused by hair in the fluid in a dot-dash pattern.

Solid Ovarian Tumours

Although rare, they are important to identify because 65 % of solid ovarian tumours are found to be malignant [2].

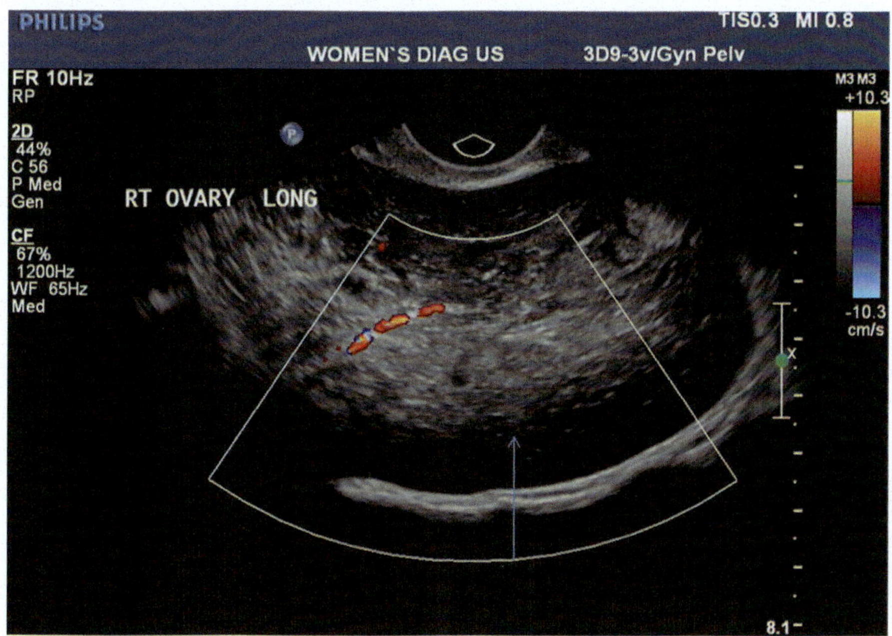

Fig. 7.23 Image of an ovary with a fibroma (solid ovarian tumour)

Figure 7.23 shows a solid mass with heterogenous echotexture. Colour Doppler imaging shows the presence of vessel within the mass. The walls are smooth. There is posterior acoustic attenuation (blue arrow). The patient underwent surgical excision and pathology showed a fibroma, which is a benign solid ovarian tumour.

Hydrosalpinx

A hydrosalpinx occurs as a result of tubal blockage. This may be due to endometriosis, infection or adhesions. Hydrosalpinx can be asymptomatic but may be a cause of infertility.

Figure 7.24a, b shows a thin-walled tubular structure, filled with anechoic fluid. There is a crescent of normal ovary (yellow arrow). Other features are the incomplete septa (blue arrows) and complete septa within the dilated Fallopian tube. The ipsilateral ovary should be clearly seen and separate from this structure.

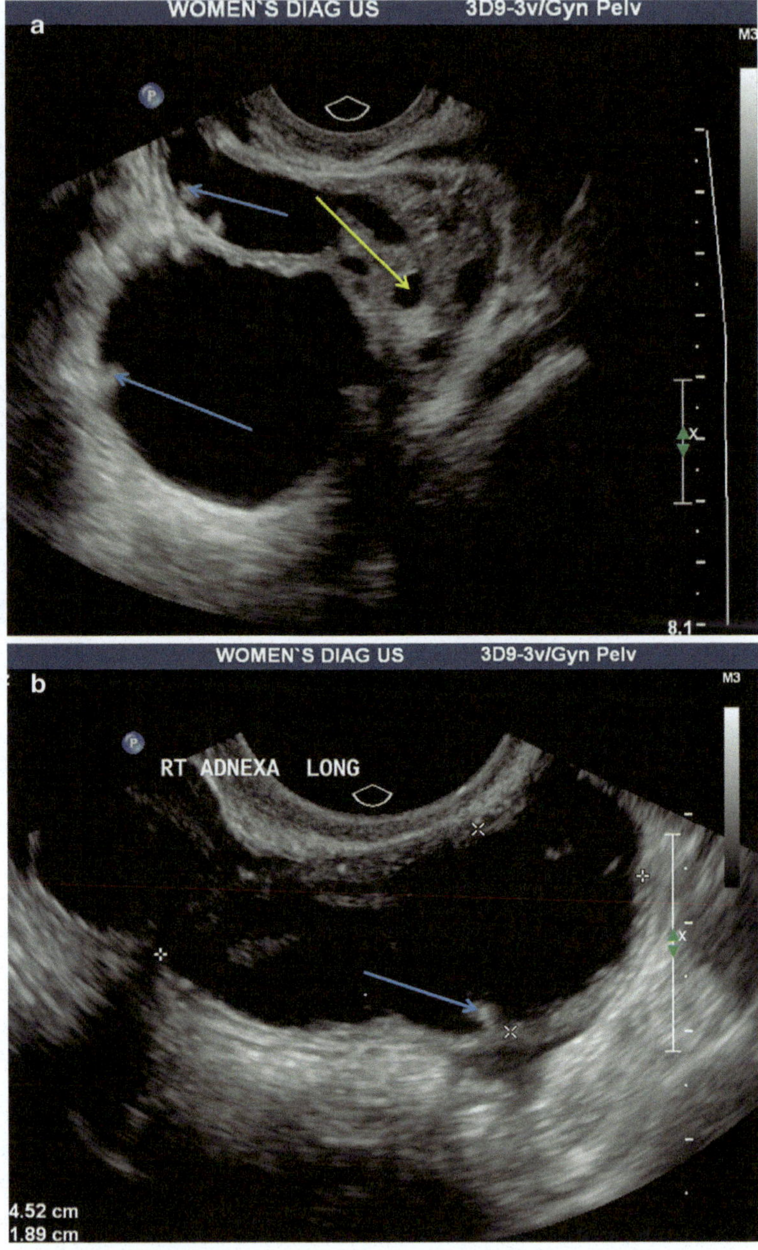

Fig. 7.24 (**a**, **b**) Hydrosalpinx

References

1. Timmerman D, Testa AC, Bourne T, Ameye L, Jurkovic D, Van Holsbeke C, Paladin D, Van Calster B, Vergote I, Van Huffel S, Valentin L. Simple ultrasound-based rules for the diagnosis of ovarian cancer. Ultrasound Obstet Gynaecol. 2008;31(6):681–90.
2. Revised 2003 consensus on diagnostic criteria and long-term health risks related to polycystic ovary syndrome. The Rotterdam ESHRE/ASRM-Sponsored PCOS Consensus Workshop Group. Fertility and Sterility, vol 81. No. 1. Jan 2004.

Chapter 8
Endoanal Ultrasound of Pelvic Floor

Peter Stewart

Anal ultrasound has been performed since 1987. It uses a modified technique developed for trans-rectal ultrasound.

Indications

1. Evaluate anal sphincter defects during investigation of faecal incontinence
2. Evaluate perianal sepsis
3. Local staging of anal and low rectal neoplasia.
4. Trans-anal biopsy of anorectal lesions

Equipment

Endoanal ultrasound for evaluation of anorectal disease is often performed using an endocavity transducer with an element that rotates 360° radially allowing circumferential assessment of the sphincteric complex (Fig. 8.1). Older machines were only two dimensional but newer models have 3-D capability (Figs. 8.2 and 8.3) as well as colour Doppler and are useful for mapping anal sphincter defects, fistula tracks and extent of neoplastic spread in cases of anorectal cancer.

P. Stewart, MBBS, FRACS
Department of Colorectal Surgery, Concord Repatriation General Hospital, Sydney, Australia
e-mail: pstewart@bigpond.com.au

L. Chan et al. (eds.), *Pelvic Floor Ultrasound: Principles, Applications and Case Studies*, DOI 10.1007/978-3-319-04310-4_8

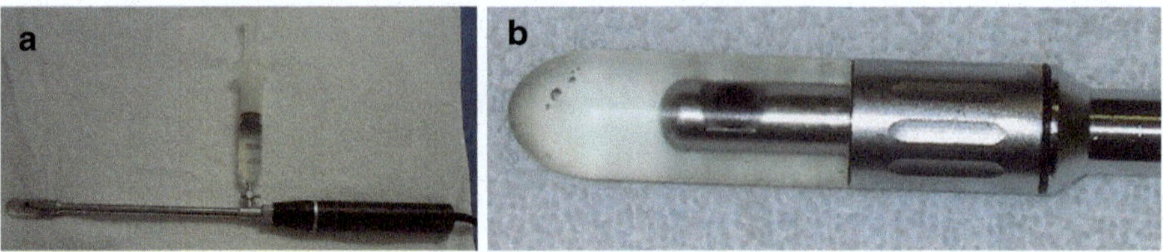

Fig. 8.1 Endocavity 2D transducer (BK 1850) with 360° rotating element (BK6005) in Hardcone for endoanal ultrasound

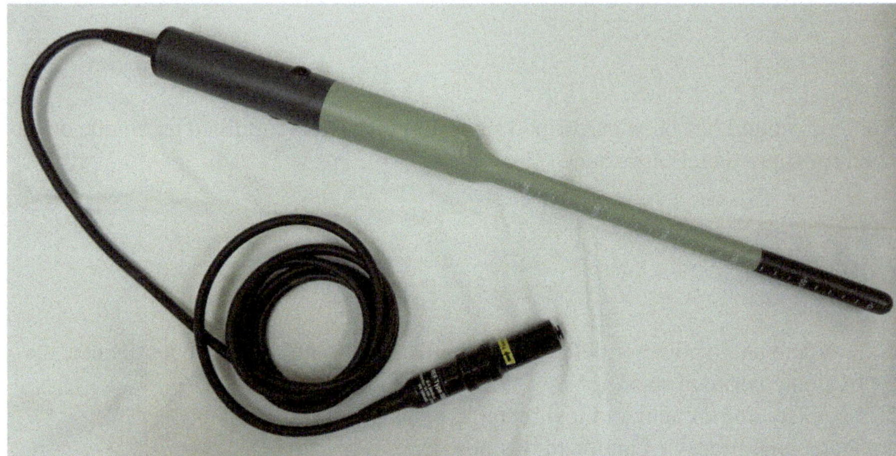

Fig. 8.2 3D endoanal transducer (BK 2052)

Technique of Endoanal and Endorectal Ultrasound

No oral bowel preparation is required. For endorectal ultrasound, a Fleet or similar enema is given just prior to the examination. No sedation or anaesthetic is needed.

Patients are positioned in the left lateral position with the buttocks close to or overhanging the edge of the examination bed. For endoanal ultrasound, the lubricated transducer is inserted a distance of about 8 cm. In the male, the distal prostate should be visualised; in the female, the cervix. Images are then obtained at the level of the puborectalis muscle, upper, mid- and lower anal canal (Figs. 8.4, 8.5, 8.6, and 8.7).

For endorectal ultrasound, the transducer is introduced to just proximal to the pelvic floor then the balloon is partly inflated with degassed water. The transducer can then be slowly manoeuvred proximally to the desired level. Alternatively the transducer can be introduced through a rigid sigmoidoscope.

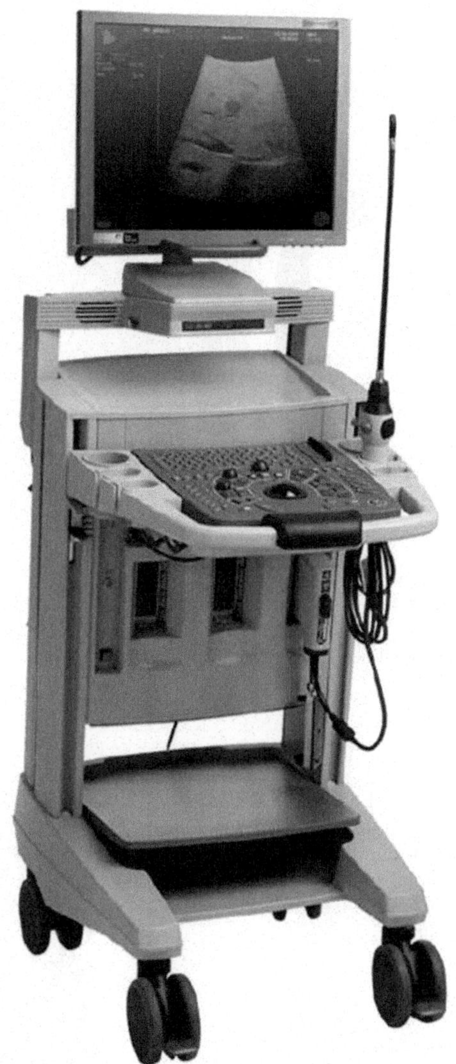

Fig. 8.3 BK Pro Focus 2202 ultrasound system

Anatomy (Fig. 8.4)

The anal canal is usually examined at four levels (Figs. 8.5, 8.6, and 8.7):

Levator ani
Upper anal canal
Mid anal canal
Distal (lower) anal canal.

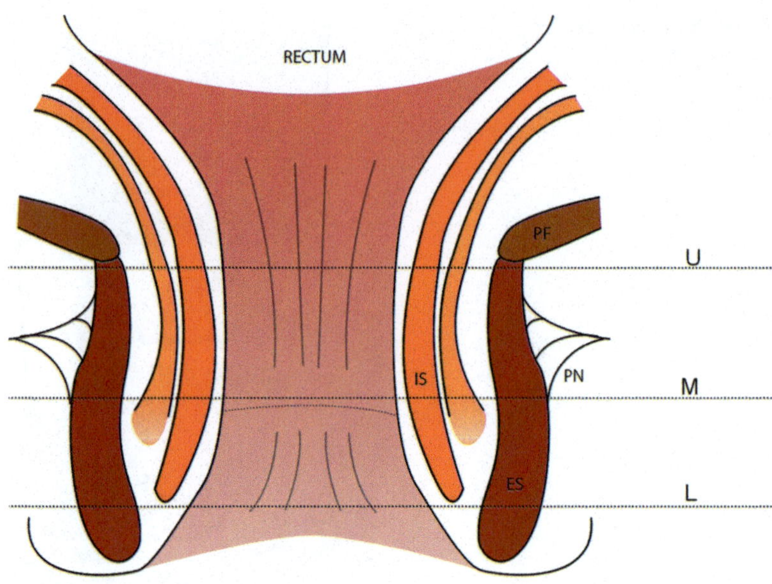

Fig. 8.4 Endoanal ultrasound- the sphincter is imaged at three levels (*upper*, *mid* and *lower levels* Figs. 8.5, 8.6 and 8.7) *ES* external sphincter, *IS* internal sphincter, *PF* pelvic floor/puborectalis, *PN* pudendal nerve

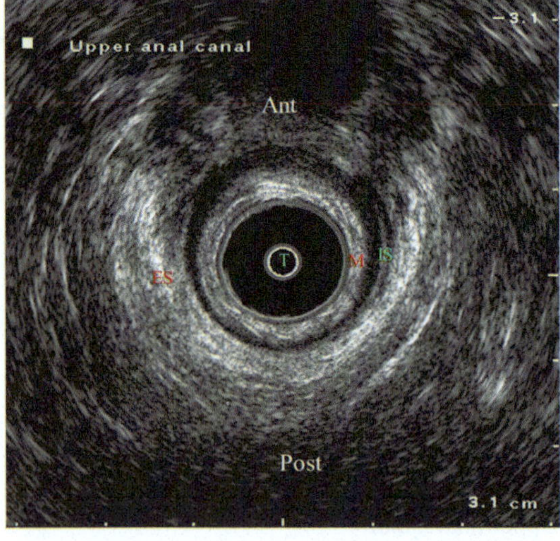

Fig. 8.5 Endoanal ultrasound image at level of upper anal canal *T* transducer, *M* mucosa, *IS* internal sphincter, *ES* external sphincter, *Ant* anterior, *Post* posterior

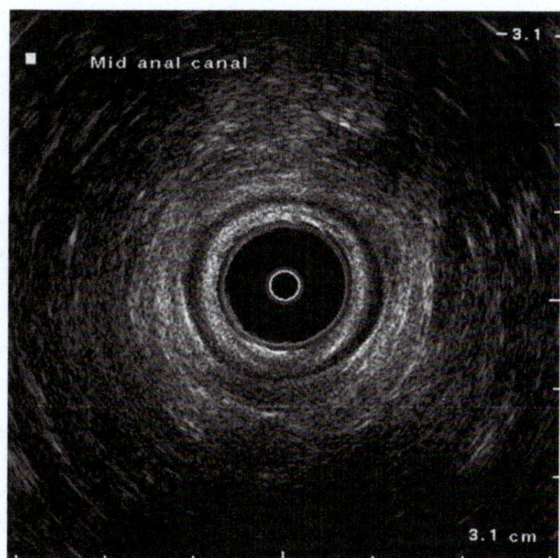

Fig. 8.6 Endoanal ultrasound image at level of mid anal canal

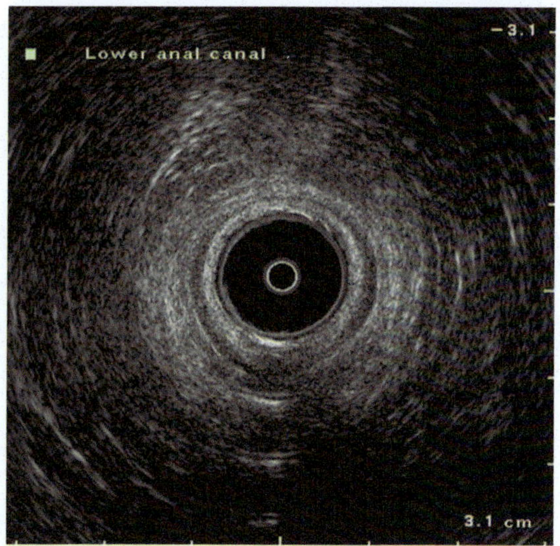

Fig. 8.7 Endoanal ultrasound image at level of distal anal canal

Indications for Endoanal Ultrasound

Evaluation of Sphincter Defects

Endo anal ultrasound is invaluable in evaluation of sphincter defects in patients with fecal incontinence. Sphincter defects may involve the internal sphincter, external sphincter or a combination. Most are obstetric related but may be traumatic (usually post surgical) or sepsis related. Defects may be discrete or multiple. Figure 8.8

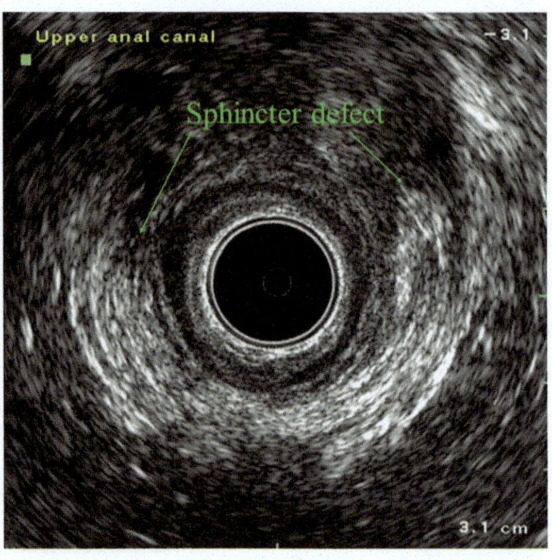

Fig. 8.8 Anterior external sphincter defect. Discrete separation of external sphincter fibres anteriorly (*arrows*) following obstetric injury and third degree tear

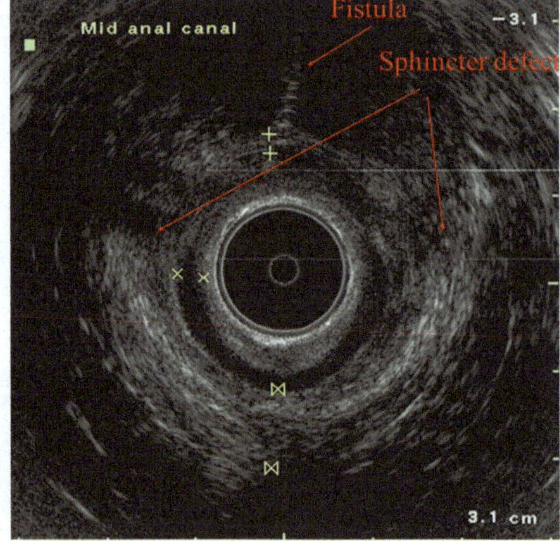

Fig. 8.9 Combined anterior internal and external sphincter defects with ano-vaginal fistula. Obstetric injury with fourth degree tear. *Arrow* shows the 'ring-down' artifact indicating air in the fistula tract

illustrates an anterior external sphincter defect following obstetric injury and third degree tear. There is discrete separation of external sphincter fibres anteriorly. Severe pelvic floor injury during delivery can result in fourth degree tears and development of ano-vaginal fistula (Fig. 8.9). Endoanal ultrasound can be helpful following surgical treatment (Figs. 8.10, 8.11, and 8.12) and in assessment of rectal prolapse (Fig. 8.13).

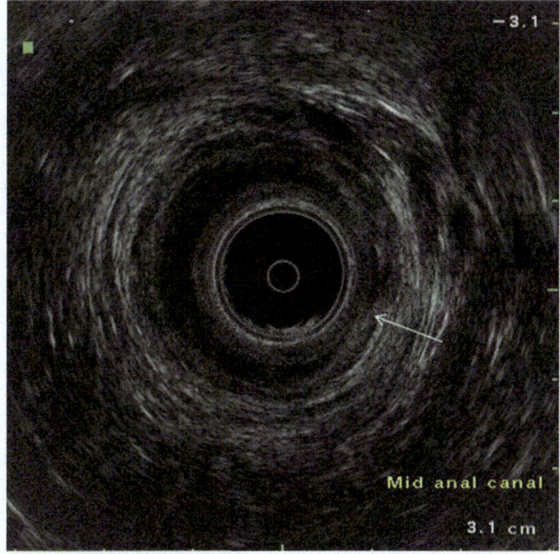

Fig. 8.10 Lateral internal sphincterotomy. The distal fibres of the internal sphincter have been surgically divided to treat fissure in ano (*arrow*)

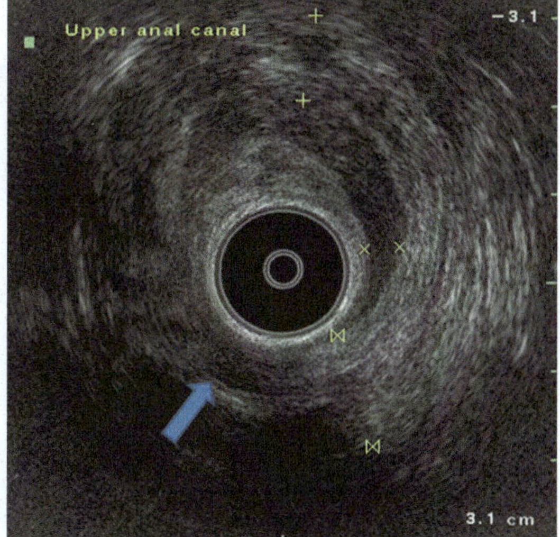

Fig. 8.11 Combined right posterior internal and external sphincter defect (*arrow*) post fistulotomy

Evaluation of Perianal Pain and Sepsis

Ultrasound can be used to evaluate obscure anal pain and identify pathologies such as occult intersphincteric abscess (See Cases 1 and 2). In patients with fistula-in-ano, ultrasound may detect the internal opening of a fistula (Fig. 8.14) and confirm the

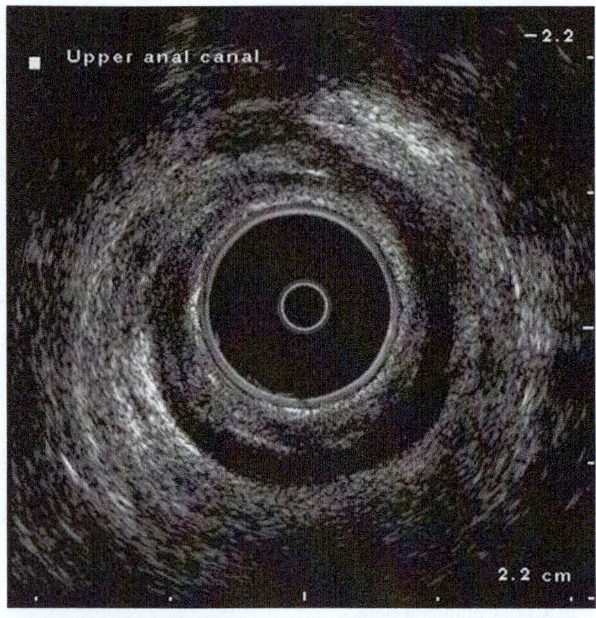

Fig. 8.12 Appearance after overlapping sphincter repair

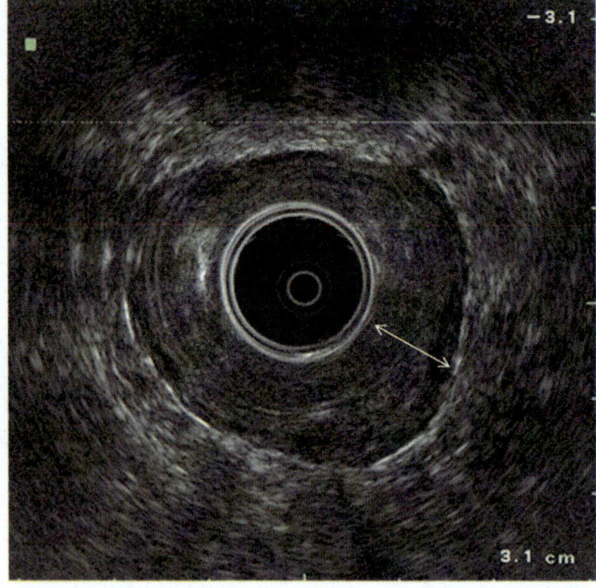

Fig. 8.13 Thickened rectal mucosa (*arrow*) consistent with full thickness rectal prolapse (about 8mm in this patient. Normally 2–3mm)

trans-sphincteric nature of the fistula track (Fig. 8.15). An appreciation of the amount of sphincter contained by the fistula can be determined. The use of 3D ultrasound allows a measurement of the proportion of involved muscle (See Chap. 9). Spread of

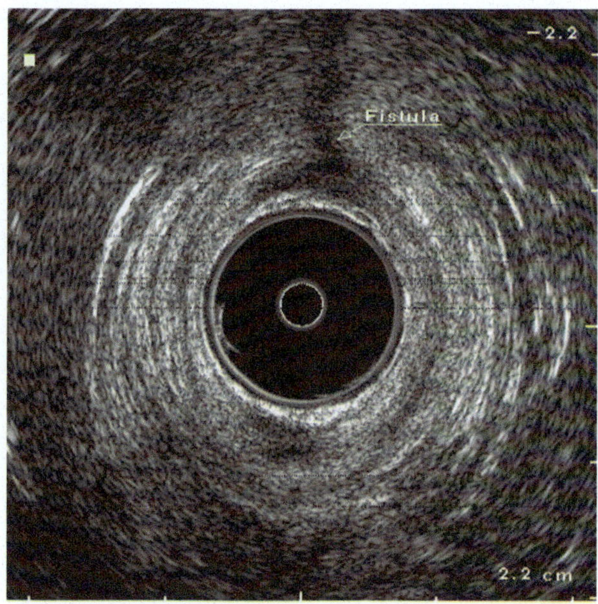

Fig. 8.14 Anterior trans-sphincteric fistula (*arrow*)

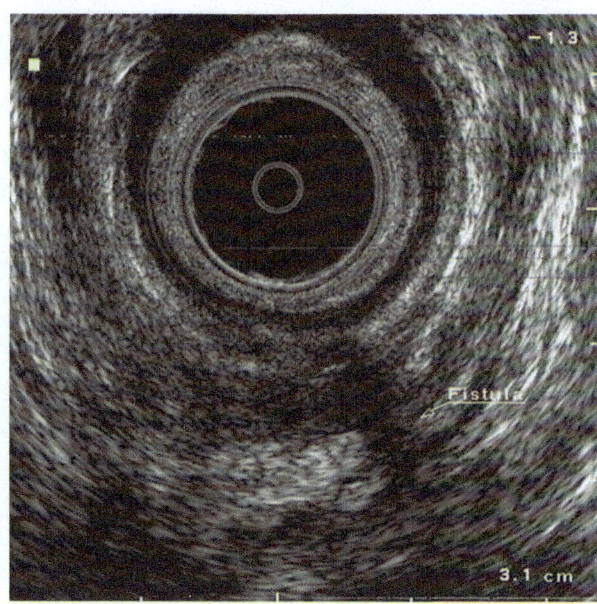

Fig. 8.15 Left postero-lateral trans-sphincteric fistula

sepsis through the perianal tissues can be demonstrated on ultrasound, allowing planning for adequate drainage and treatment. Figure 8.16 demonstrates a posterior abscess cavity and Fig. 8.17 shows a horseshoe abscess.

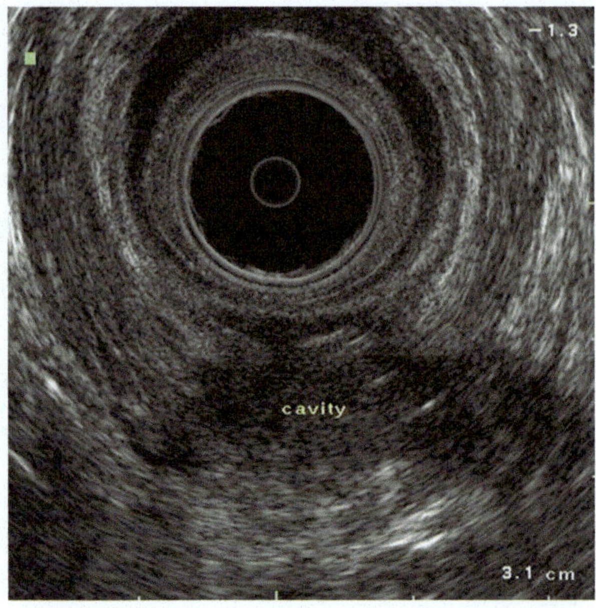

Fig. 8.16 Deep posterior abscess cavity

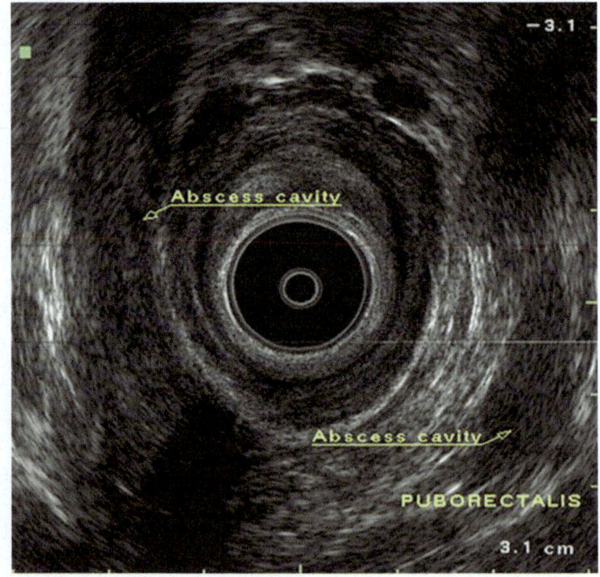

Fig. 8.17 Horseshoe abscess

Case 1

Male age 42 presented with over 12 months of dull anal pain. The pain was present constantly, a little worse on opening his bowels. There was no PR bleeding nor change in bowel habit. He was otherwise well.

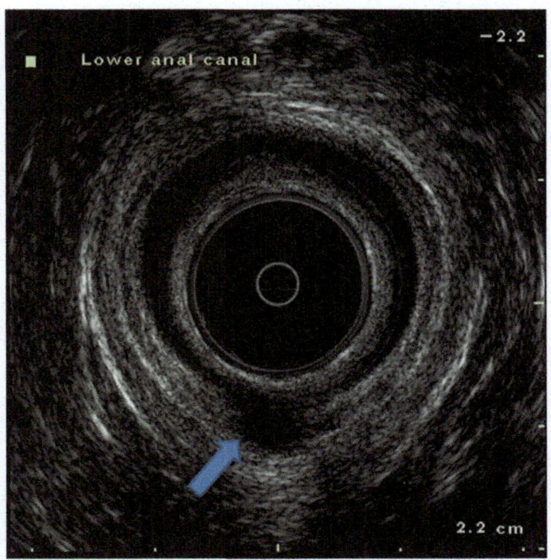

Fig. 8.18 Small posterior intersphincteric abscess (*arrow*)

Physical examination showed no obvious perianal pathology. No fissure or fistula identified. There was slight tenderness posteriorly on digital examination of the anal canal.

Ultrasound revealed a small posterior intersphincteric abscess (Fig. 8.18). The abscess was drained via a small posterior intersphincteric incision. A 1 cm diameter 'mass' of granulation tissue was removed. The patient had an uneventful recovery with remission of symptoms.

These abscesses are thought to develop due to infection of a small anal crypt gland which passes into the intersphincteric plane where it becomes trapped.

Case 2

A 56 year old male presented with 18 months of chronic anal pain. The pain was constant, dull, worse at night and slightly worse with opening bowels. No bleeding or change in bowel habit. Physical examination revealed a tender mass posteriorly in the distal rectum. There was no anal tenderness.

Ultrasound revealed a 30×20 mm hypoechoic mass posterior to the rectum. An opening into the upper anal canal can be seen in this view (Fig. 8.19a, b).

This is an intersphincteric abscess which has tracked cranially above the sphincters to lie behind the rectum. It is usually drained by passing a probe through the internal opening directed cranially and then laying open the posterior rectal wall. The patient made an uneventful recovery.

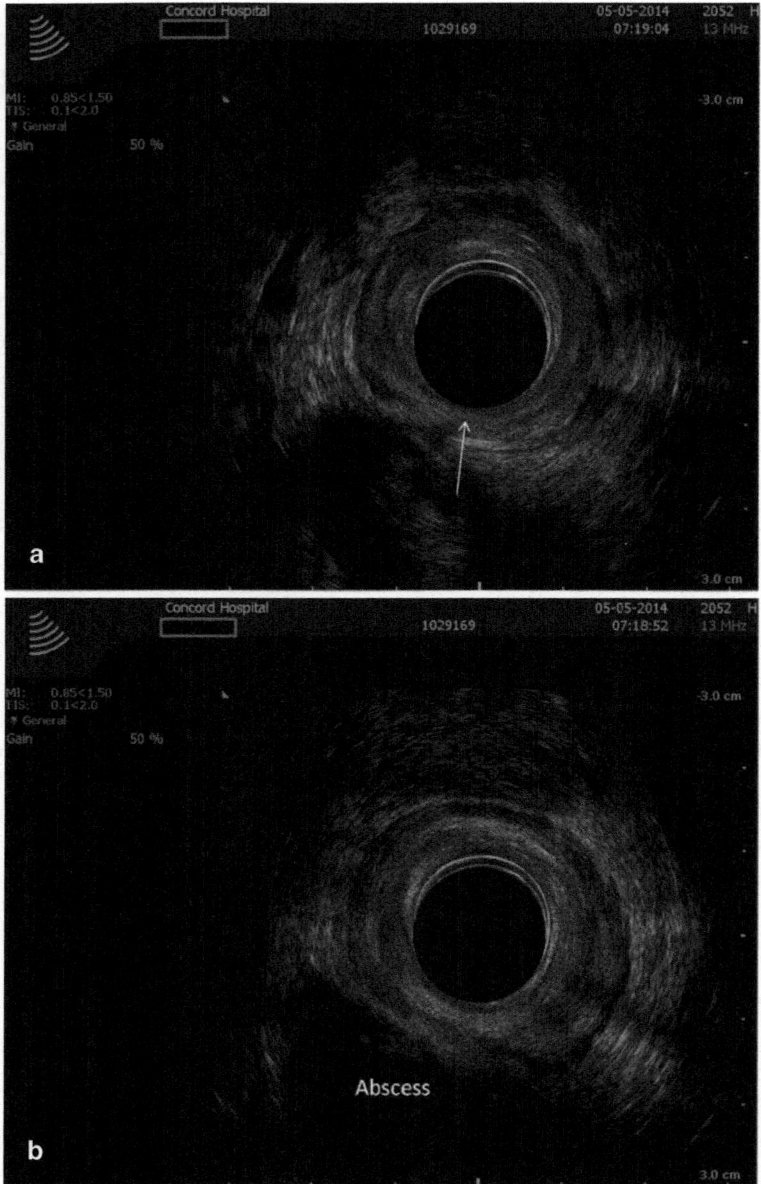

Fig. 8.19 (**a**) Large chronic retrorectal abscess with opening into upper anal canal (*arrow*). (**b**) Same patient demonstrating large retrorectal component of the hypoechoic abscess cavity

Local Spread of Ano-rectal Tumours

Ano rectal ultrasound allows pre-operative T and N staging of ano-rectal malignancy. This assists with pre-operative decision making (local excision vs radical resection; pre-operative radiotherapy; involvement of adjacent tissues)

Case 3

Seventy-one year old male who had ultra-low anterior resection 2 years prior for Stage II adenocarcinoma of distal rectum. Presented with asymptomatic recurrence found at routine follow-up colonoscopy. The patient was unable to have a staging MRI scan due to cardiac pacemaker in situ.

Transrectal Ultrasound with an endocavity sector end-fire transducer shows absence of plane between tumour and prostate (Fig. 8.20). There was no metastatic disease. This patient underwent pelvic exenteration (cystoprostatectomy and abdomino-perineal excision of rectum) with curative intent.

Case 4

Male age 71. Previous high anterior resection 18 months earlier for Stage I adenocarcinoma of proximal rectum. Routine follow-up CT showed lesion in posterior mesorectum 10 cm from anal verge. The lesion was glucose avid on PET scan. The patient underwent transrectal ultrasound guided core biopsy (Fig. 8.21a, b) which showed metastatic prostate cancer and was commenced on androgen deprivation therapy.

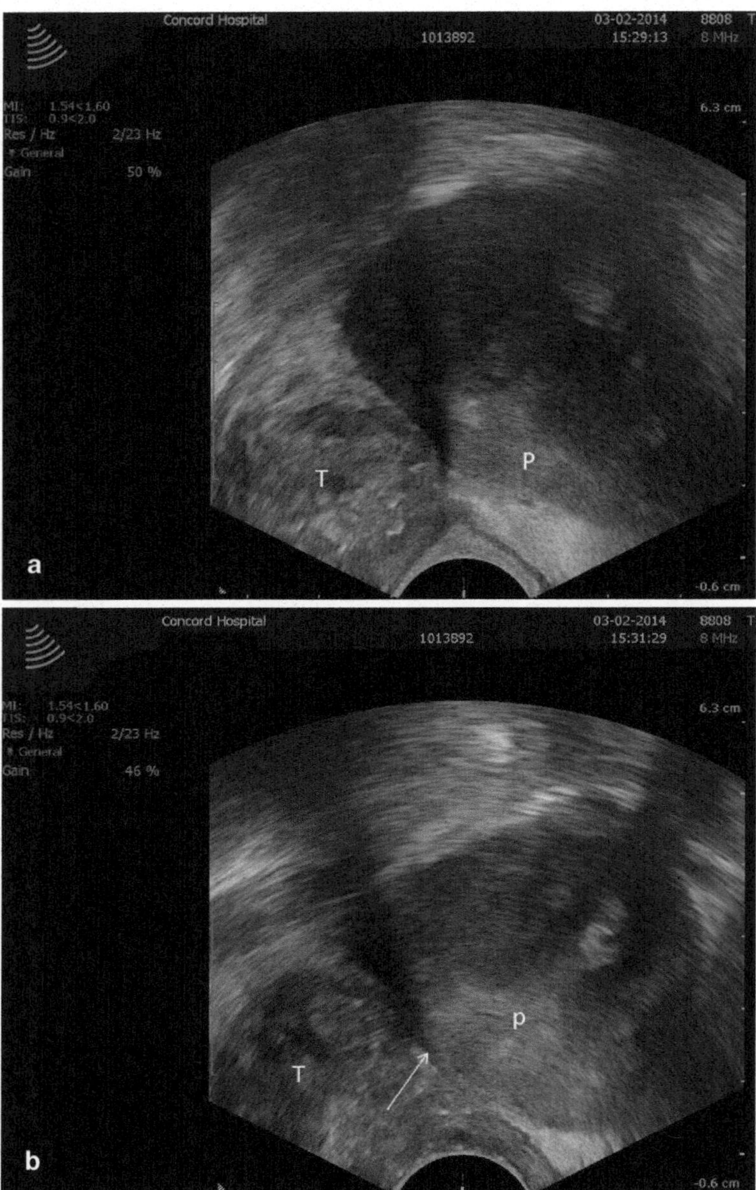

Fig. 8.20 (**a**) Recurrent adenocarcinoma of distal rectum (*T*) adjacent to prostate (*P*). (**b**) Endoanal ultrasound with end-fire transducer showing absence of clear plane (*arrow*) between tumour and prostate

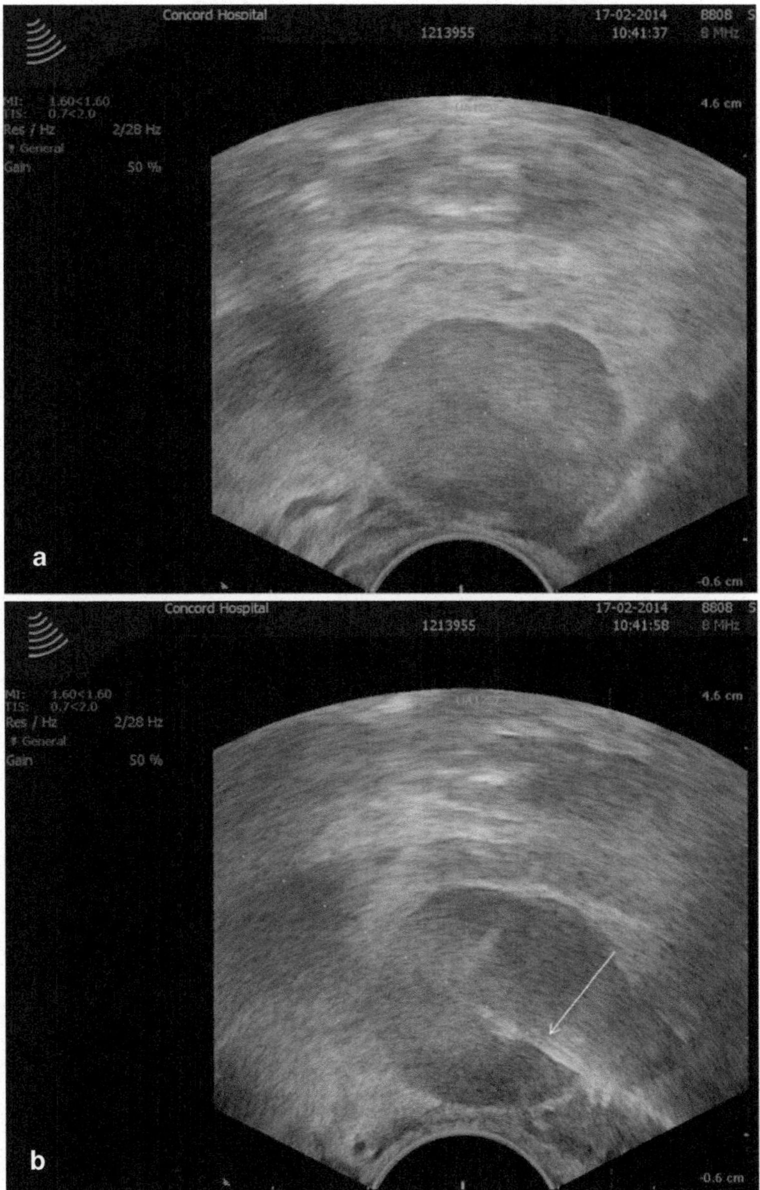

Fig. 8.21 (**a**) Sagittal image of mass in posterior mesorectum (*T*) obtained using end-fire transducer. (**b**) Transrectal ultrasound guided core biopsy (*arrow*) showed metastatic prostatic cancer

Chapter 9
Principles and Applications of 3D Pelvic Floor Ultrasound

Shelley O'Sullivan, Vincent Tse, Stephanie The, Lewis Chan, and Peter Stewart

3D pelvic floor ultrasound imaging has an emerging role in the assessment and management of pelvic floor disorders. Whilst many patients with voiding dysfunction, incontinence and pelvic organ prolapse can be assessed utilizing dynamic 2D imaging as shown in the previous chapters, there is increasing interest in the use of 3D/4D ultrasound imaging in complex pelvic floor dysfunction. Furthermore, advances in ultrasound equipment and transducer technology has brought this modality within reach of many clinicians.

Potential applications of 3D ultrasound in pelvic floor dysfunction include assessment of sling and mesh complications, pelvic organ prolapse, obstetric pelvic floor injuries, fecal incontinence and complex perianal sepsis/fistulae.

S. O'Sullivan, RDMS
Ultrasound, Philips Healthcare Australia, Epping Road, North Ryde, NSW 2113, Australia
e-mail: shelley.osullivan@philips.com

V. Tse, MBBS, MS, FRACS • L. Chan, MBBS(Hons), FRACS, DDU (✉)
Department of Urology, Concord Repatriation General Hospital, Sydney, NSW, Australia
e-mail: vincent.tse@sydney.edu.au; lewis.chan@sswahs.nsw.gov.au

S. The, MBBS, FRANZCOG, DDU, COGU
Department of Women's and Children's Health, Pelvic Floor Unit, Westmead Hospital, Sydney, NSW, Australia
e-mail: wdu@optusnet.com.au

P. Stewart, MBBS, FRACS
Department of Colo-Rectal Surgery, Concord Repatriation General Hospital, Sydney, NSW, Australia
e-mail: pstewart@bigpond.com.au

L. Chan et al. (eds.), *Pelvic Floor Ultrasound: Principles, Applications and Case Studies*, DOI 10.1007/978-3-319-04310-4_9

Principles of 3D Ultrasound

With 3D ultrasound imaging a series of sagittal images (or axial images in some endocavity 360° transducers – see Case 4) are collected which make up a volume data set (Fig. 9.1a, b). This can then be manipulated and reconstructed in different planes to obtain extra information not easily available from 2D imaging. The acquisition of a 3D volume dataset can be automated within the mechanics of the 3D transducer (either mechanical or electronic steering of the ultrasound beam) or less commonly by freehand movement (a 'sweep') of the transducer.

2D greyscale ultrasound imaging allows the operator to image the organ or region of interest in two planes (the sagittal and transverse planes). The ability to acquire a 3D ultrasound dataset (volume) allows reconstruction of the axial plane which is generally not able to be obtained in 2D imaging. This process is called multi-planar reconstruction, similar to the process of reconstructing images in sagittal and coronal planes on a CT scan.

The ability to perform volume rendering allows the user to reconstruct a 3D image which may help in diagnosis. There are also powerful algorithms that allow real-time updating of the 3D reconstructed image, producing a so-called '4D' capability (the fourth dimension being time). These processes require considerable computing/post-processing of the echo information and together with the physical limits of ultrasound (e.g. Pulse repetition frequency, field of view, lines of sight, etc. – see Chap. 1) can lead to lower resolution of the reconstructed image.

Technique of 3D Volume Acquisition and Analysis

3D Definitions and instrumental controls:

Pixel – A term used to describe the basic unit of 2D information displayed on an ultrasound image. Each pixel is assigned a series of gray scale X and Y Values.

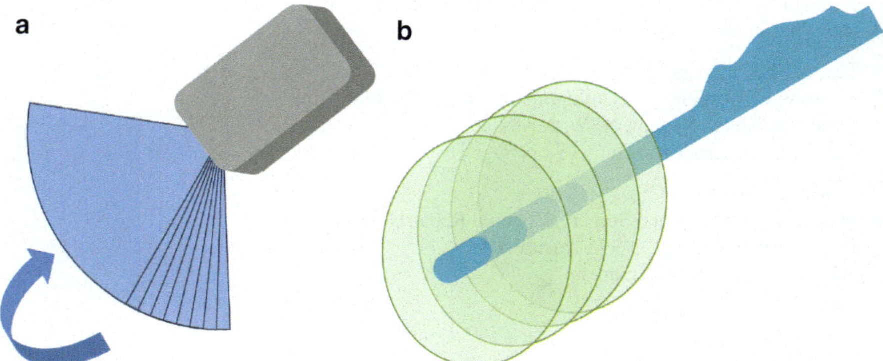

Fig. 9.1 (**a, b**) 3D volume acquisition. A series of sagittal (**a**) or axial (**b**) images are acquired by the transducer to obtain a 3D volume dataset

Voxel – A term used to describe the basic unit of 3D information, as it has an additional vector of Z attached to it, to specify its location in the 3D volume. It is assigned the same series of gray scale values X, Y and the additional Z.

MPR (Multi planar reconstruction – Figs. 9.2 and 9.3) – MPR consists of the three planes that make up the 3D data set. They are positioned 90° from each other and

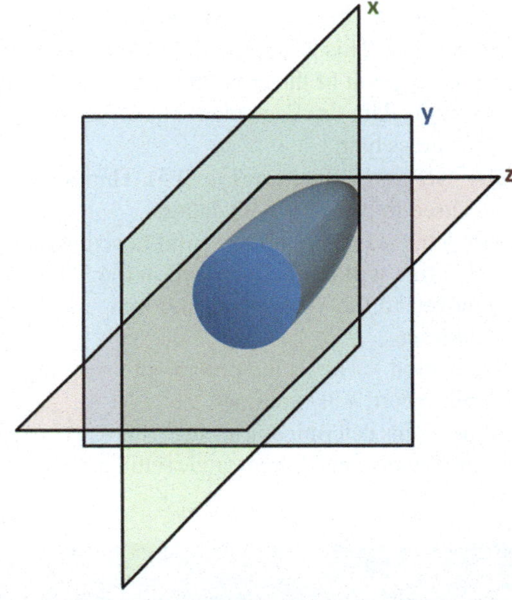

Fig. 9.2 Multiplanar reconstruction – the 3D ultrasound volume dataset can be analysed by manipulating the three planes (X, Y, Z) at right angles to each other

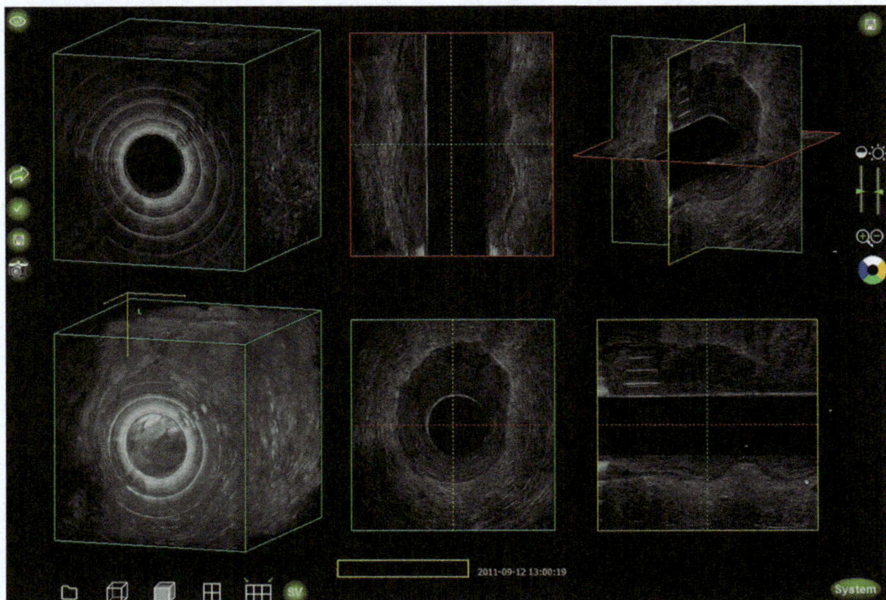

Fig. 9.3 MPR – 3D volume obtained by endoanal 3D transducer

labeled X, Y and Z. When one plane is manipulated, the other planes on view will change accordingly. Figure 9.4 illustrates the three MPR planes during 3D volume analysis. By convention the top left box is the acquisition plane, which is the sagittal plane in the example. This is the plane that was used initially to acquire the data set. The top right box is the orthogonal view to the acquisition plane. In the above case it's the transverse view. The bottom left box is the coronal or C-plane view which is derived from the combination of acquisition and orthogonal views. This is the plane which is not generally possible on 2D imaging.

Cross Hair – This is a marker of the intersection of each plane (Fig. 9.4). The intersecting point of the cross hair on each view represents the same point within the volume data set. Each plane rotates around the corresponding line that makes up the cross hair.

ROI – Region of Interest (Fig. 9.5). This is the user defined area on 2D imaging that is used to produce a 3D data set.

Trim Line – In Fig. 9.5 the solid horizontal line is the trim line. Anything above this line will not be included in the 3D data set. Therefore, this line should be moved to the very top of the image so that information is not cut out of the data set.

Acquisition – This is the process of sweeping, pivoting or performing live 2D that will record a 3D volume.

Angle – This determines the range (thickness of the 3D volume) over which the acquisition will occur. Larger angle settings results in a larger volume acquired (Fig. 9.6).

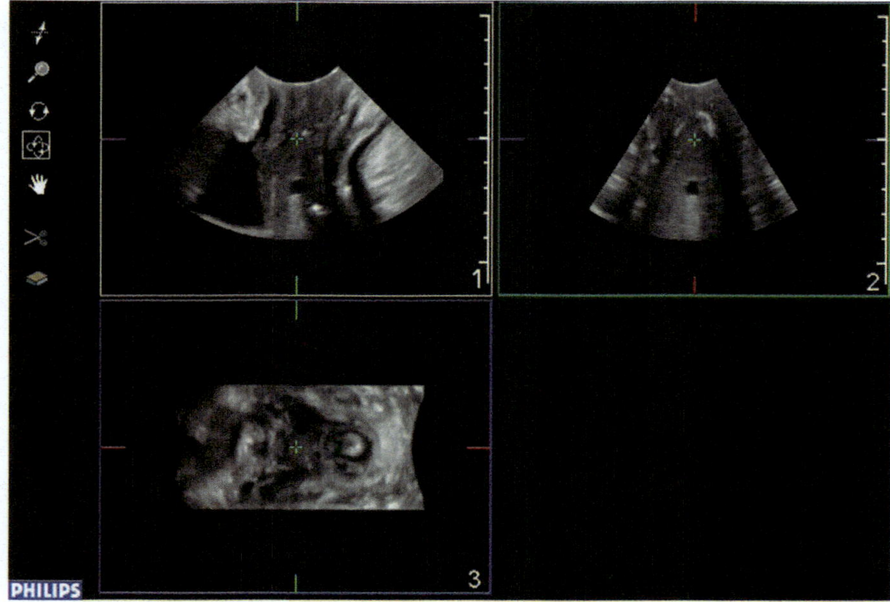

Fig. 9.4 Cross hair – this is a marker of the intersection of each plane. The intersecting point of the cross hair on each view represents the same point within the volume data set

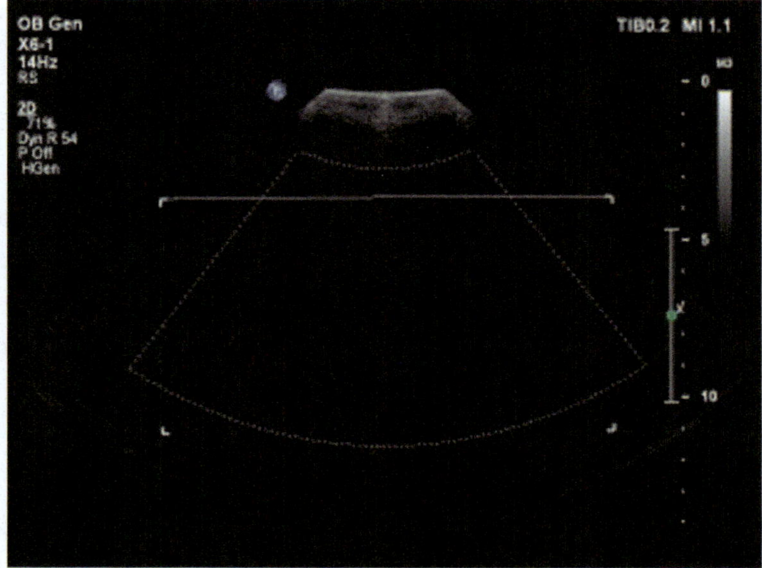

Fig. 9.5 Region of Interest (ROI). This is the user defined area on 2D imaging that is used to produce a 3D data set. The *white triangular* shaped area is the ROI box

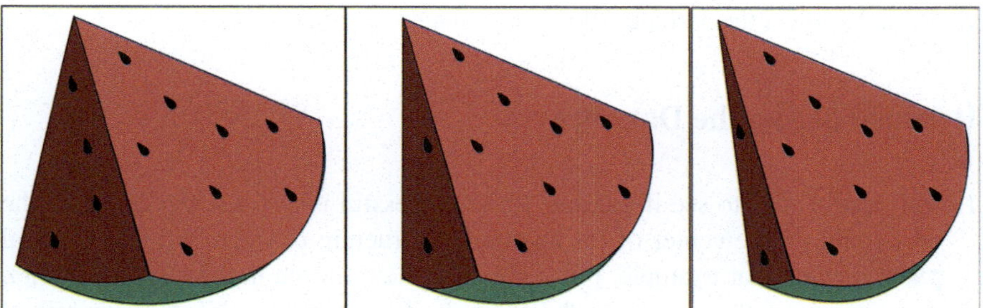

Fig. 9.6 Sweep angle – this determines the range (thickness of the 3D volume) over which the acquisition will occur

Technique of 3D Data Acquisition (See Tips 9.1)

1. Obtain the best 2D image possible. In pelvic floor transperineal imaging this is achieved in the mid-sagittal plane. It is important to ensure there is adequate sonographic gel and enough pressure on the transducer to maintain good contact with the perineum and eliminate any air between the transducer and the perineum.
2. Initiate the 3D process.
3. Expand the ROI box (Fig. 9.5) to its maximum position to encompass the entire area of interest.
4. Increase the sweep angle (Fig. 9.6). If the region of interest is large (such as the pelvic floor) larger angles are required to capture the entire area.

Tips 9.1 How to Acquire Good 3D Images
Technique of acquiring 3D volume datasets during transperineal imaging

- The results of 3D data analysis depend on the quality of image data acquired
- A high quality 2D image acquisition will allow good 3D data capture
- Use the same gain adjustments (TGC, LGC, Gain, ROI) settings to optimize image before performing 3D acquisition
- Keep patient relaxed and comfortable to minimize unintended pelvic floor activation especially in assessment of pelvic organ prolapse
- Use lots of sonographic gel and ensure good contact between perineum and transducer (but not excessive pressure to distort anatomy)
- Start in mid-sagittal plane

5. Centre the ROI in the 2D image. For transperineal pelvic floor imaging it is helpful to use the urethra, vaginal canal or rectum as central landmarks. Obtain the best 2D image of the urethra, bladder, rectum, and vaginal canal as possible.
6. Activate the 3D sweep to capture the volume data.
7. Save the data set once this has been acquired making sure that it is the entire data set and not just the 3 plane-MPR image that is saved.

Reconstructing the Data Set

1. The easiest way to see if the data set is successful is to place the center of the cross-hairs in the center of the anatomical structure of interest (in the sagittal plane image). For example, place the cross hairs in the middle of the urethra, sling, mesh or anorectum. In the example dataset in Fig. 9.7, the suburethral sling will be used as the structure of interest. If the image is clearly defined in each of the three MPR views then a data set has been acquired that can successfully be manipulated.
2. If the data set is usable then select the top left box for manipulation. Selecting an individual box on the MPR view allows manipulation of that particular view in all directions X, Y and Z. The top left box of the MPR data set is the acquisition plane. This is the plane used initially to acquire the data set. Manipulating the X, Y and Z planes will manipulate the view so that it is in the exact location to display the structures of interest. Manipulating the X plane while still in the acquisition plane will rotate the image like a rolodex (eg. elongate the urethra in this particular view to obtain a true sagittal section- Fig. 9.8).
3. Manipulating the Y plane will sweep the transverse image from the left arm of the sling to the right arm of the sling in the acquisition plane (like a revolving door) (Fig. 9.9). While manipulating the Z plane will cartwheel the image (Fig. 9.10).

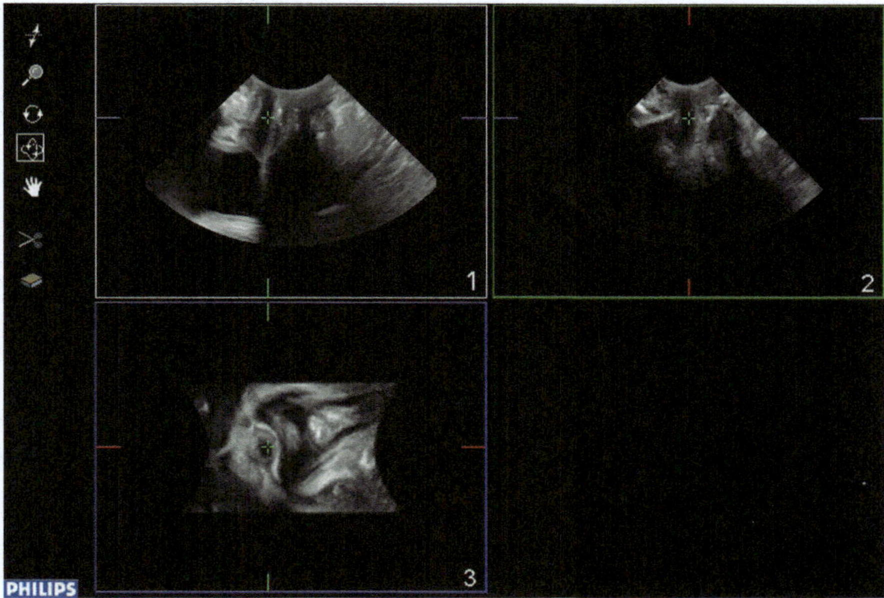

Fig. 9.7 A usable 3D volume dataset obtained by transperineal ultrasound of patient with mid-urethral sling – the image is clearly defined in each of the 3 MPR views

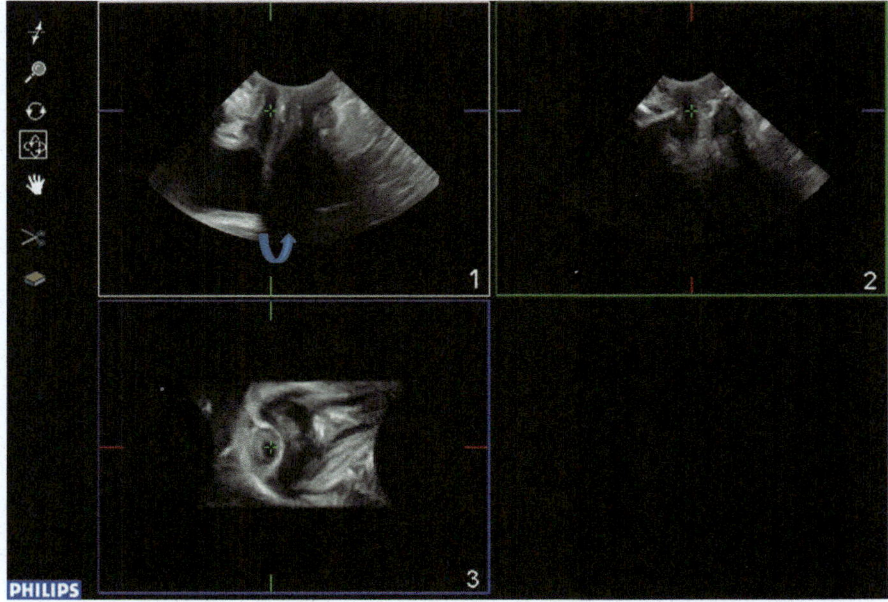

Fig. 9.8 MPR – manipulating the X plane. This will rotate the image like a rolodex (*arrow*), elongating the urethra in this particular view to obtain a true mid-sagittal section

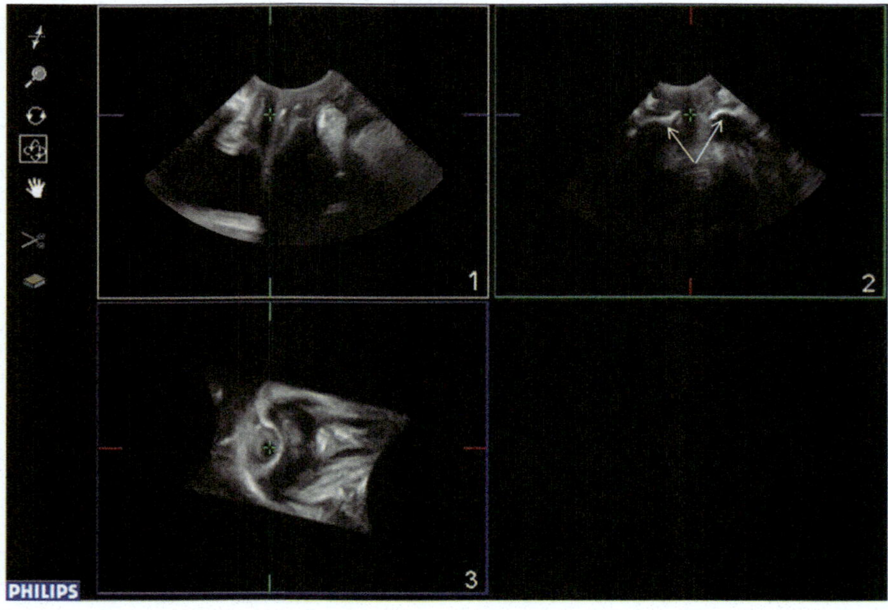

Fig. 9.9 MPR – manipulating the Y plane. This will sweep the transverse image from the left arm of the sling to the right arm of the sling (*arrows*) in the acquisition plane (like a revolving door)

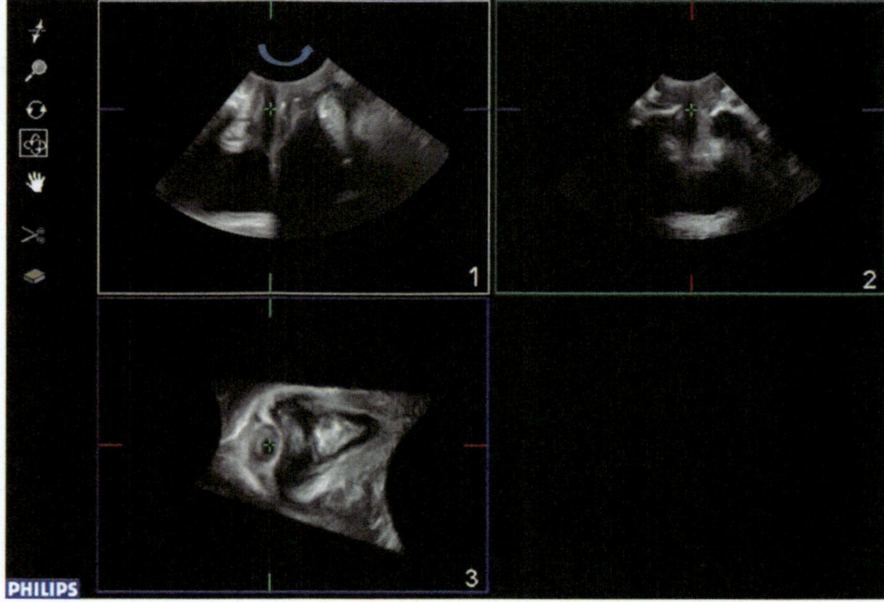

Fig. 9.10 MPR – manipulating the Z plane will cartwheel the image (*arrow*)

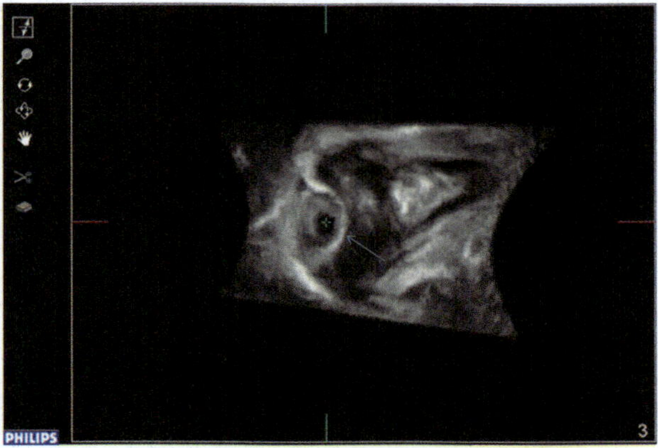

Fig. 9.11 Manipulating the coronal image so that both arms of the sling (*arrow*) are clearly displayed

4. Then select the transverse view (the top right box) for manipulation. Only minimal manipulation is needed. Move the X, Y and Z plane individually to produce the desired image. The pelvic floor should have a similar appearance on both sides of the midline of the image.
5. Once the sagittal and transverse planes have been adjusted successfully the coronal (axial) plane is where most of the manipulation will occur. Place the cross hairs on or at the level of the base of the sling.
6. Select the coronal plane (bottom left box) and then select the control button that changes the view setting to a single image (the coronal view) instead of the three views. This will allow a single (the coronal image) to be captured and fine adjustments to be performed. Then remove the cross hairs to ensure the image is free of obstructions.
7. Continue to manipulate the data using the X and Y plane controls to obtain the desired image (eg. manipulating the X plane will allow inclusion of both arms of the sling in the image. Manipulating the Y plane will rotate the image to adjust how much of the arms of the sling are visible (Fig. 9.11).
8. Capture the coronal image.

Case 1 Persisting Voiding Dysfunction Post Sling Division

A 52 year old female presents having underwent excision of a suburethral segment of sling for voiding difficulties following a synthetic mid urethral sling. Urodynamics showed poor flow with protracted void and elevated voiding pressures. Postoperatively she had only mild improvement and complained of persisting symptoms of poor flow and incomplete bladder emptying. Transperineal 3D ultrasound scan was performed to assess residual sling position (Fig. 9.12).

Comments – (Also See Chap. 5) The differential diagnosis of persisting symptoms post treatment of voiding dysfunction due to an obstructive sling procedure

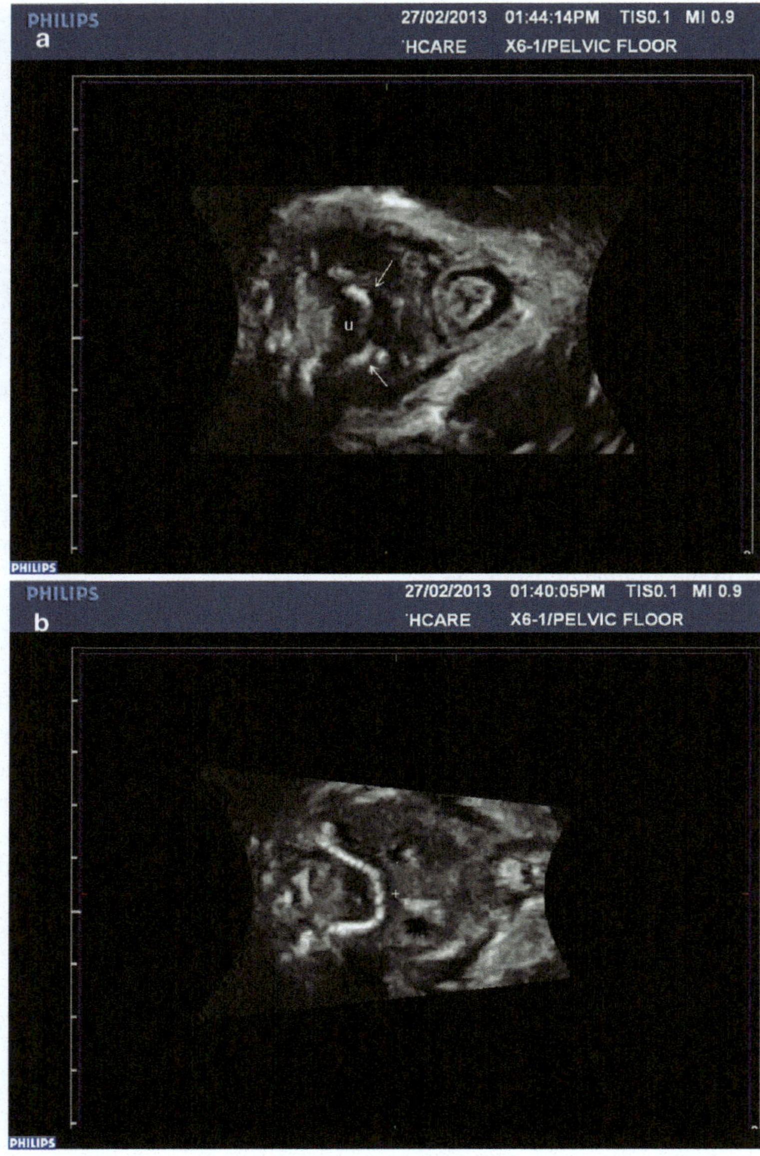

Fig. 9.12 (**a**, **b**) Transperineal 3D ultrasound images in patient with persisting voiding dysfunction post sling division demonstrating insufficient division of the sling (*arrows*) with a segment of sling continuity (**b**)

include residual/recurrent obstruction or hypocontractile (underactive) bladder. 3D ultrasound can be used to assess the adequacy of sling division. The images (Fig. 9.12a, b) showed there was insufficient division of the sling with a segment of sling continuity. The patient underwent re-exploration and excision of the residual sub-urethral mesh segment.

Figure 9.13 demonstrates a patient who had recurrence of voiding dysfunction 6 months following sling division. The X-plane image showed the effect of scar contraction with insufficient separation of the sling segments following simple division of the obstructive sling. This patient subsequently underwent re-exploration and excision of a sub-urethral segment of sling.

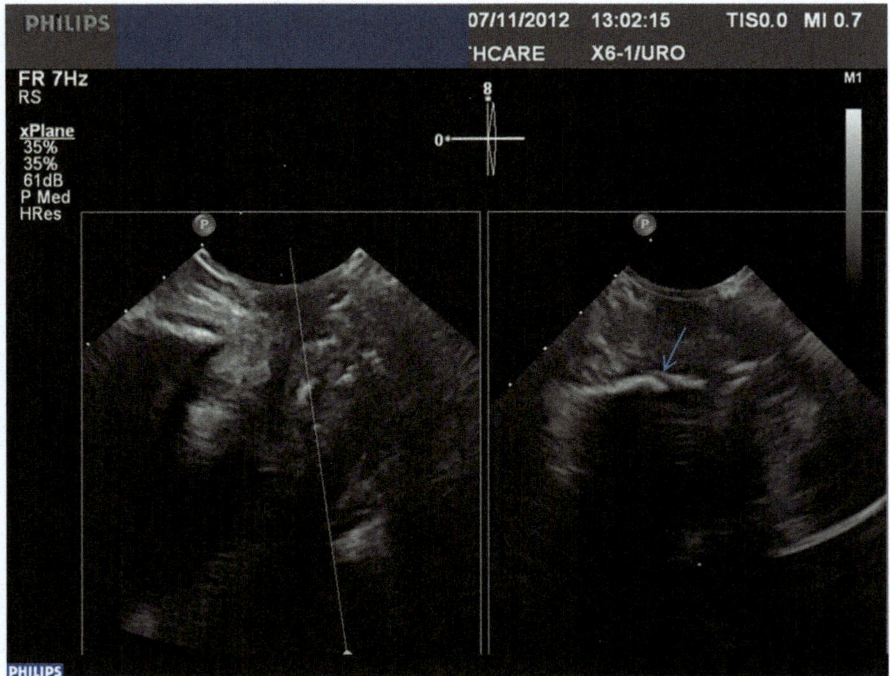

Fig. 9.13 Recurrent voiding dysfunction post sling division – the X-plane (transverse) image (*right image*) shows the effect of scar contraction with insufficient separation of the sling (*arrow*) segments following division of the obstructive sling

Case 2 Persisting Incontinence Despite 2 Sling Procedures

A 47 year old female presents with persisting urinary stress incontinence despite the placement of a transobturator mid urethral sling, and subsequent placement of another synthetic mid-urethral sling. 3D pelvic floor ultrasound scan was performed to assess sling positions.

The image (Fig. 9.14) shows the value of 3D Pelvic floor ultrasound in identification of sling location relative to the urethra in complex cases where there is prior sling surgery especially in planning further treatment. The two slings have been placed in the same position. Urodynamic study demonstrated intrinsic sphincteric deficiency with low leak point pressures and little urethral mobility (see Chap. 5). The patient subsequent underwent excision of the suburethral portions of the slings and placement of a pubo-vaginal fascial sling at the level of proximal urethra.

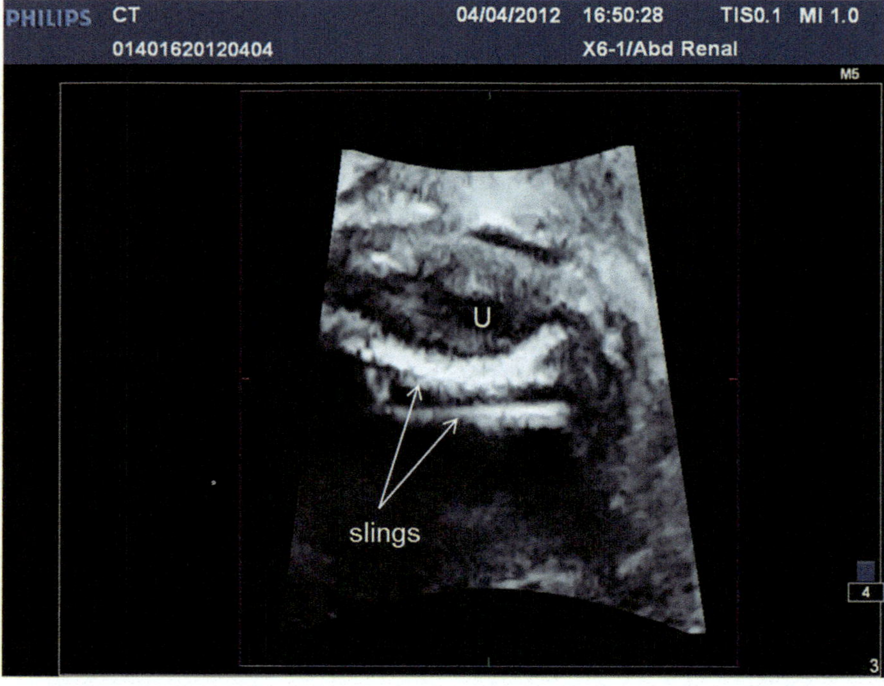

Fig. 9.14 Persisting incontinence despite two slings. The ultrasound image showed that the two slings have been placed in the same position at level of mid urethra

Case 3 Dysuria and Hematuria, Previous Sling and Bulking Agent

A 75 year old female presents with dysuria and two episodes of macroscopic haematuria. She had a background of a transobturator mid urethral sling procedure that did not improve her incontinence She subsequently underwent two injection procedures of a bulking agent (Macroplastique), which eventually improved her urinary continence. Cystoscopy showed urethral erosion of the injectable implant at the level of proximal urethra. Transperineal 3D pelvic floor ultrasound was performed to further evaluate the extent of the synthetic injected material which extended from proximal to mid urethra adjacent to the sling (Fig. 9.15).

Comments The images showed the Macroplastique (silicone microspheres) material, which is typically quite echogenic. The implant extended from proximal to mid urethra adjacent to the sling and is best appreciated on the axial reconstruction (Z plane) in Fig. 9.16.

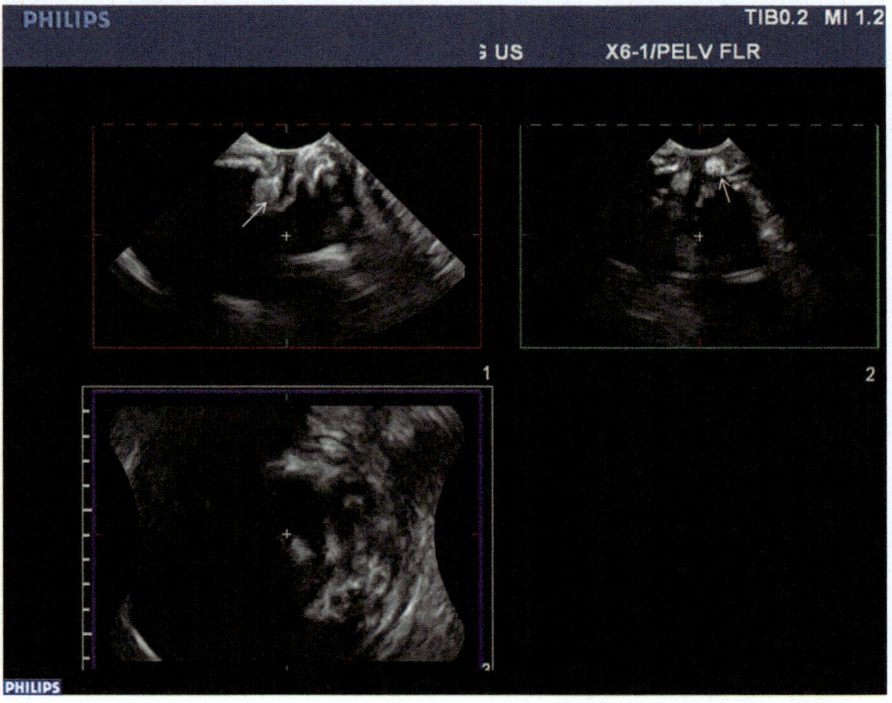

Fig. 9.15 MPR view of patient with a mid-urethral sling and injection of bulking agent. The Macroplastique® implant is echogenic and can be seen in the sagittal and transverse planes (*arrows*)

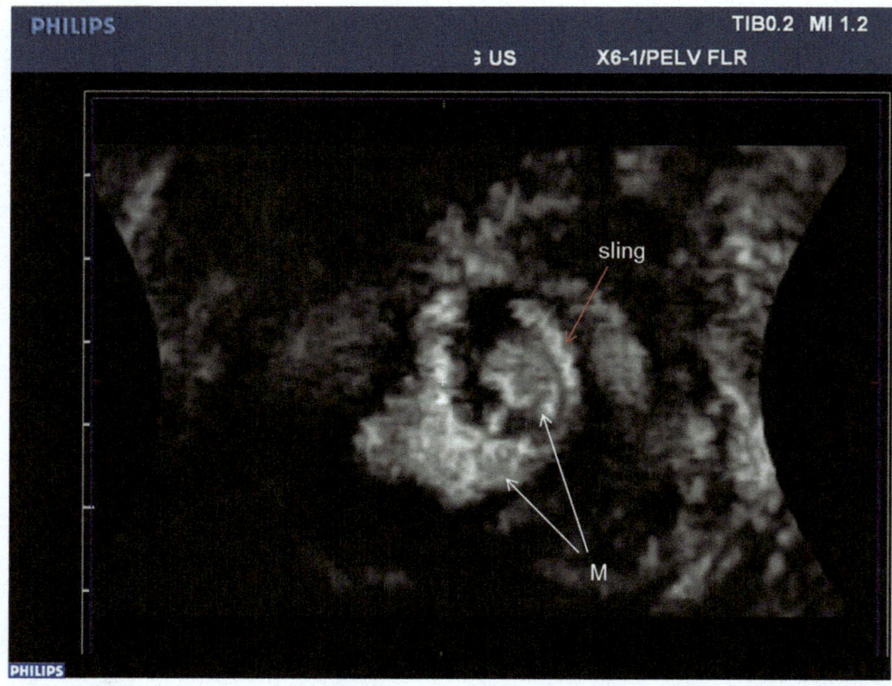

Fig. 9.16 Axial reconstruction demonstrating the Macroplastique® bulking agent (*M*) and the mid-urethral sling

The patient eventually decided to continue an expectant approach as she was reluctant to undergo further surgery to remove the implant due to the likelihood of requiring urethral reconstruction, possible fascial sling procedure and the risk of developing a fistula.

Case 4 Chronic Anal Pain, Intersphincteric Fistula

A 55 year old female presented with 12 month history of chronic anal pain. There was no bleeding or alteration of bowel habits. There was mild tenderness anteriorly on right side on digital examination. The 3D endoanal ultrasound images (Fig. 9.17) showed a trans-sphincteric abscess with fistula through the lower part of the anal canal with well preserved sphincter proximal to the fistula. She underwent a LIFT (ligation of intersphincteric tract) procedure with good outcome.

Apart from assessment of ano-rectal abscess and fistulae, endoanal ultrasound with 3D reconstruction can assist in the assessment of ano-rectal malignancy both in preoperative staging and in cases of recurrent tumour following surgery.

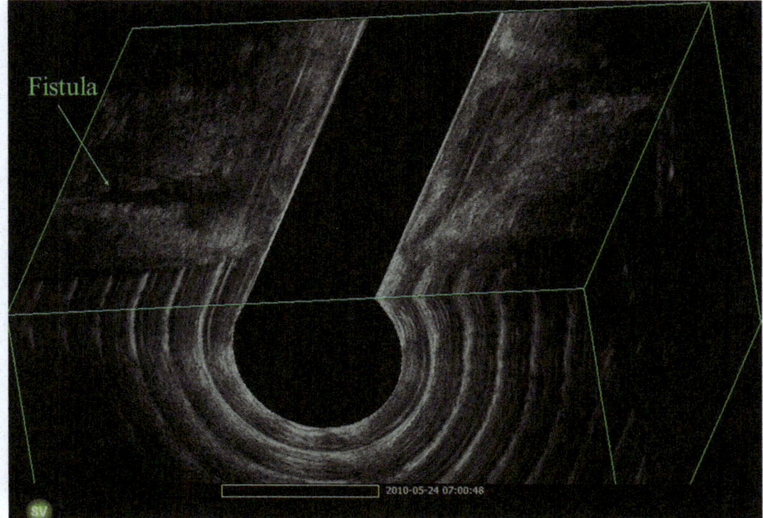

Fig. 9.17 Trans-spincteric abscess with fistula (*arrow*) through the lower part of the anal canal with well preserved sphincter proximal to the fistula

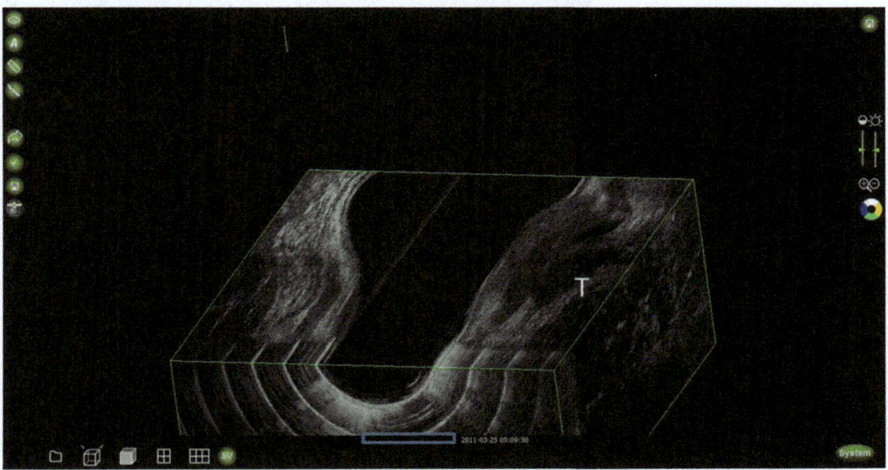

Fig. 9.18 Squamous cell carcinoma (T)

Figure 9.18 shows a reconstructed 3D image of anal squamous cell carcinoma showing extent and depth of invasion. Figures 9.19 and 9.20 are cases of locally advanced rectal carcinoma; in one case there was tumour involving the capsule of the prostate and the other shows lymph node metastases.

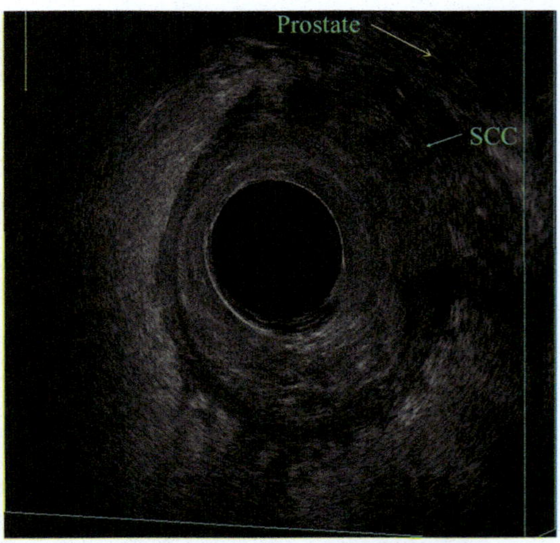

Fig. 9.19 Locally advanced rectal carcinoma involving capsule of the prostate

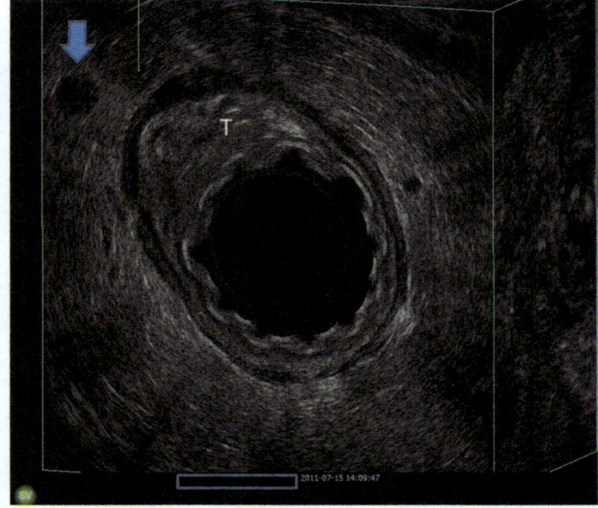

Fig. 9.20 Locally advanced rectal carcinoma (*T*) with lymph node metastases (*arrow*)

Case 5 Symptomatic Pelvic Organ Prolapse (POP)

A 61 year old lady presents with bothersome vaginal bulge symptoms. These symptoms were especially prominent at the end of a long day at work where she had to stand up for long periods of time. It was often associated with lower back pain that tended to subside when she lay down. She also complained of urinary frequency, urgency and sensation of incomplete bladder emptying. Vaginal examination revealed a POP-Q Stage 3 cystocele with associated vault prolapse.

Comments The key feature of a cystocele is its low position relative to the inferior border of the symphysis pubis, either at rest or straining. There may also be distortion of the urethra with hypermobility, bladder neck opening and rotational descent. The 3D axial images at rest and on Valsalva demonstrates descent of the cystocele with widening of the levator haitus (Figs. 9.21 and 9.22)

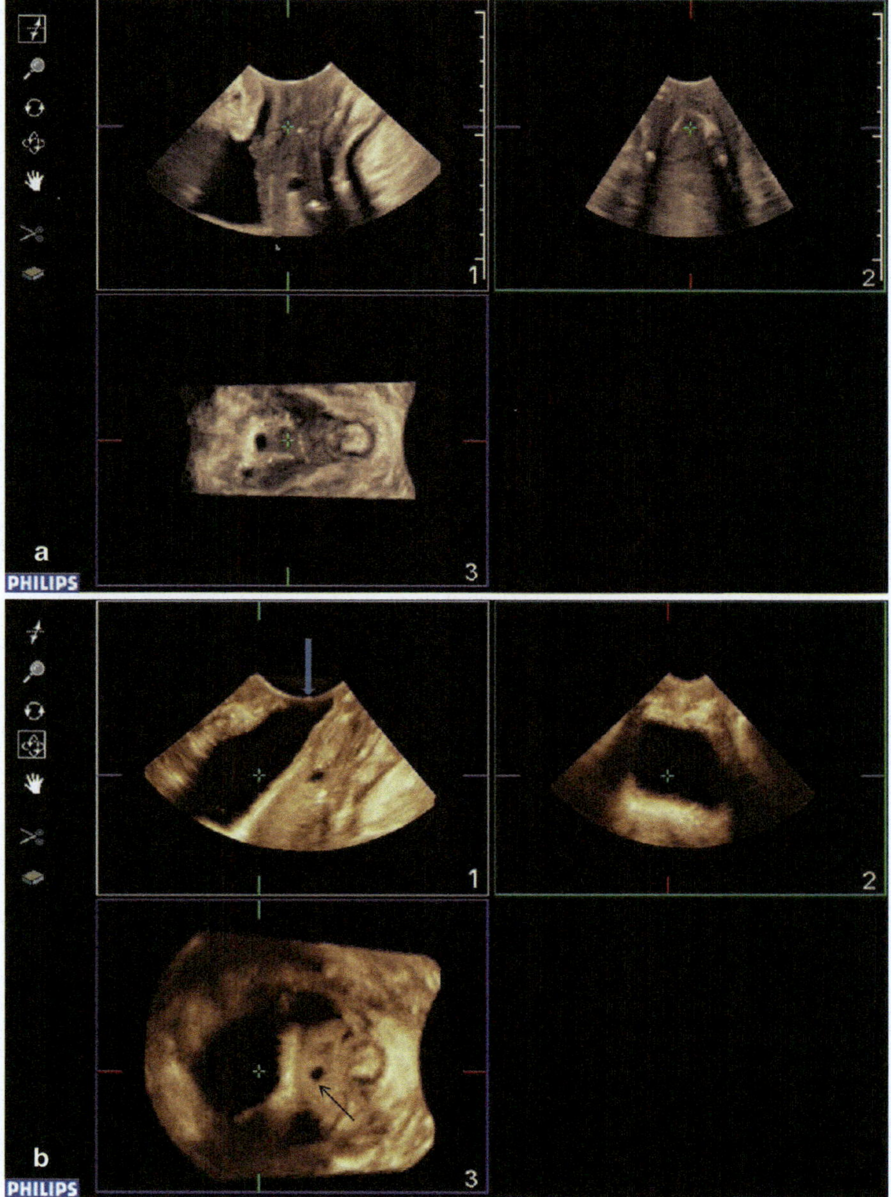

Fig. 9.21 Cystocele- 3D volume datasets with patient at rest (**a**) and on maximal Valsalva (**b**). Note Nabothian cyst in cervix seen in sagittal and axial views (*arrow*). Adjusting the display colour map such as using the 'chroma' setting in these images may assist in demonstrating some pathologies

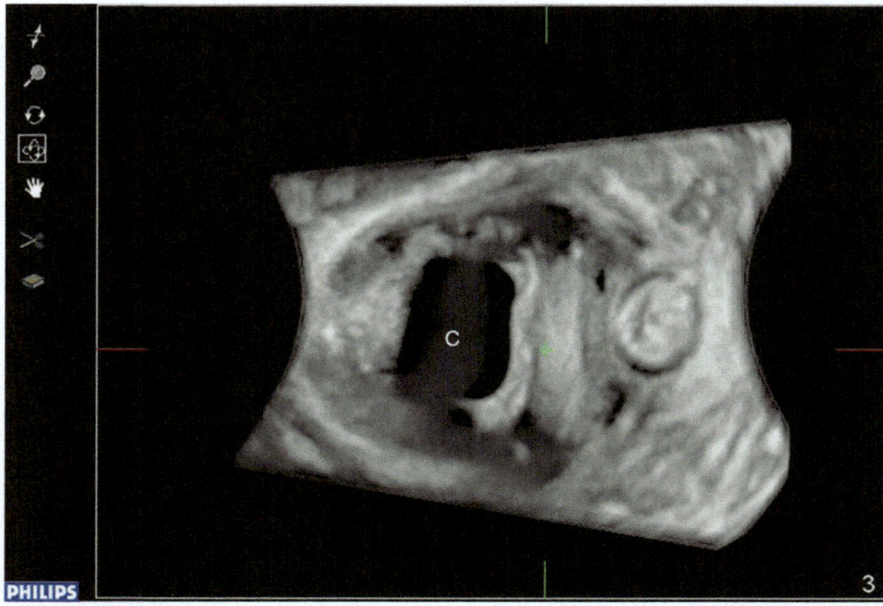

Fig. 9.22 Coronal reconstruction image of pelvic floor in patient with cystocele (*c*)

3D Pelvic Floor Ultrasound in Assessment of Pelvic Organ Prolapse

Advances in 3D ultrasound imaging has opened up new opportunities for studying the functional anatomy of the pelvic floor. 3D pelvic floor ultrasound is especially useful in the assessment of pelvic organ prolapse (POP) and can be performed by transperineal (translabial) or transvaginal approaches. Whilst POP is routinely assessed by clinical examination, 2D/3D pelvic floor ultrasound can clearly demonstrate to the pelvic floor surgeon which pelvic viscera are involved in the prolapse and the degree (stage) of prolapse. The imaging findings can add to the clinical examination findings and assist the surgeon in deciding what type of reconstruction is most suitable for the patient. Occasionally, what is seen at physical examination may represent clinical understaging (a 'false-negative') of the actual prolapse present. This is due to levator co-activation which can prevent the maximal extent of the prolapse from presenting at the bedside [1]. This phenomenon can often be seen on ultrasound and may be due to a generalized defensive reflex [2].

One of the pathophysiological factors in POP is levator avulsion (LA), thought to be predominantly related to obstetric trauma [3, 4]. 3D imaging is of particular importance in the assessment of this entity as the levator ani muscle is well demonstrated in the axial plane (Figs. 9.23 and 9.24). Dietz et al. [3] have reported in uro-gynaecological

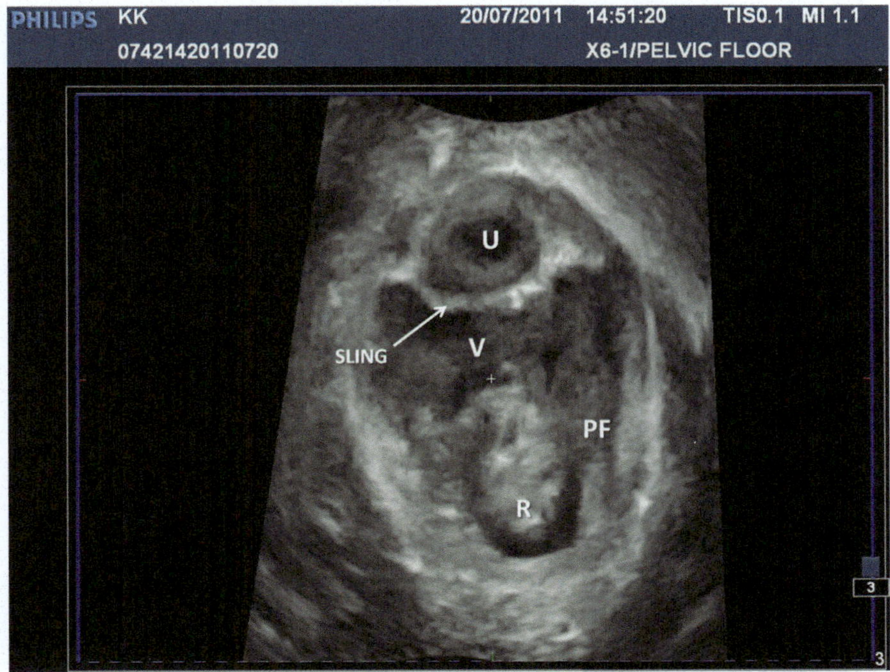

Fig. 9.23 Coronal reconstruction of pelvic floor in patient with stress incontinence cured by a mid-urethral synthetic sling. *U* urethra, *V* vagina, *R* rectum, *PF* pelvic floor muscle

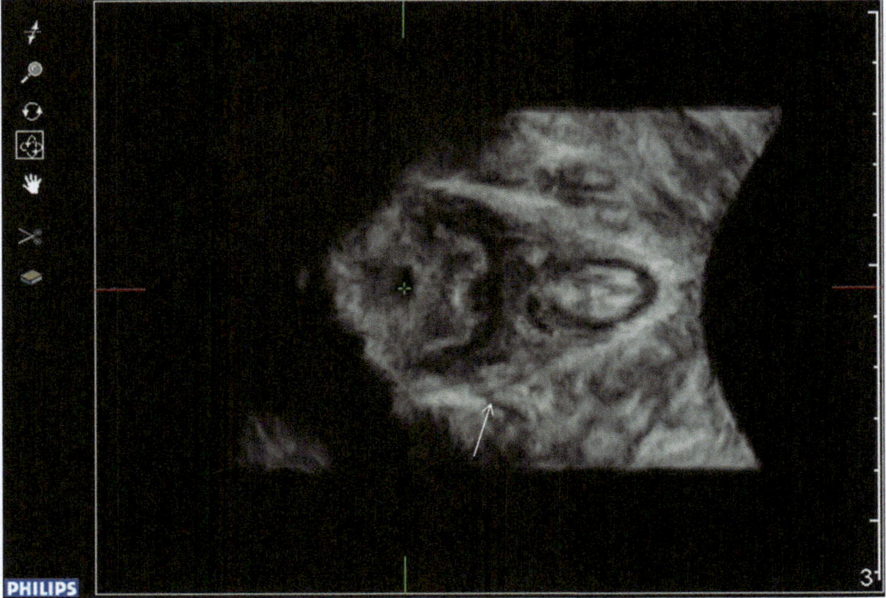

Fig. 9.24 Levator tear (*arrow*) in patient with urinary incontinence but no pelvic organ prolapse

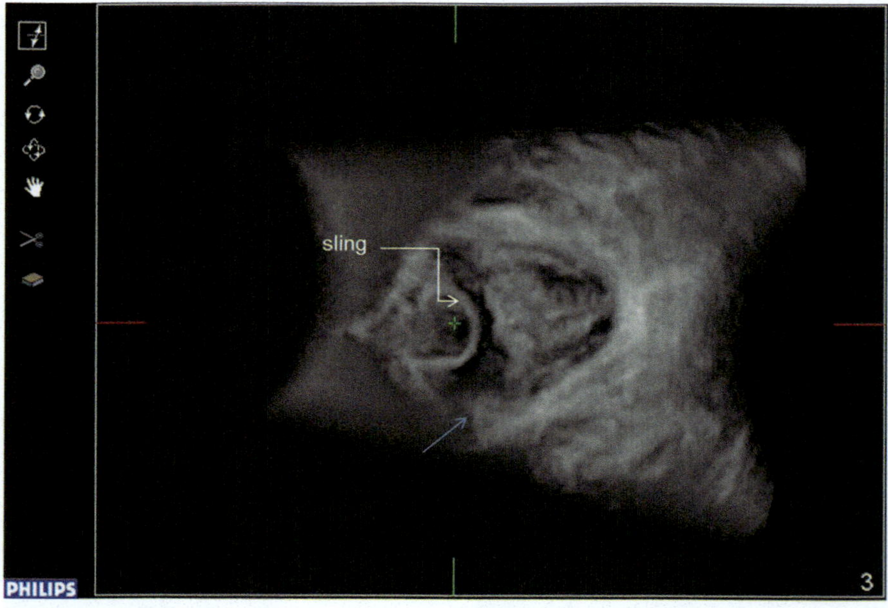

Fig. 9.25 Levator tear (*blue arrow*) with paravaginal defect in patient with stress incontinence cured by mid-urethral sling

patient cohorts that the presence of LA is associated with a twofold increased risk of Stage 2 or above POP (mainly cystocele and uterine prolapse). Furthermore when LA is identified, it is often associated with paravaginal defects and may have implications regarding surgical reconstructive approach (Fig. 9.25). Shek et al. reported that in patients undergoing native tissue cystocele repair, the presence of LA on pelvic floor ultrasound is associated with an increased risk of treatment failure/recurrence [5]. However, levator defects are not associated with urinary symptoms or voiding dysfunction [6].

3D pelvic floor ultrasound is also useful in understanding what happens when surgery fails, especially if there has been placement of synthetic meshes. Shek et al. demonstrated on 3D imaging that POP recurrence after anterior mesh reconstruction can occur dorsal to the mesh, implying dislodgement of the mesh arms [7].

If a patient presents with de novo dyspareunia after mesh repair, 3D ultrasound may also be useful in assessing the configuration and location of the mesh in addition to clinical vaginal examination. The mesh may appear crenulated and folded on ultrasound, corresponding to induration or firm bands palpable on clinical examination. Identification of such findings may reflect on technical issues during mesh placement and assist in planning surgical correction/mesh removal.

References

1. Dietz HP. Why pelvic floor surgeons should utilize ultrasound imaging. Ultrasound Obstet Gynecol. 2006;28:629–34.
2. van der Velde J, et al. Vaginismus, a component of a general defensive reaction. An investigation of pelvic floor muscle activity during exposure to emotion-inducing film excerpts in women with and without vaginismus. Int Urogynecol J Pelvic Floor Dysfunct. 2001;12:328–31.
3. Dietz HP, Simpson JM. Levator trauma is associated with pelvic organ prolapse. BJOG. 2008;115(8):979–84.
4. Steensma AB, Konstantinovic ML, Burger CW, de Ridder D, Timmerman D, Deprest J. Prevalence of major levator abnormalities in symptomatic patients with an underactive pelvic floor contraction. Int Urogynecol J. 2010;21(7):861–7.
5. Dietz HP, Chantarasorn V, Shek KL. Levator avulsion is a risk factor for cystocele recurrence. Ultrasound Obstet Gynecol. 2011;37(4):500.
6. Dietz HP, Steensma AB. The prevalence of major abnormalities of the levator ani in urogynaecological patients. BJOG. 2006;113(2):225–30.
7. Shek KL, Dietz HP, Rane A, Balakrishnan S. Transobturator mesh for cystocele repair: a short to medium term follow-up using 3D/4D ultrasound. Ultrasound Obstet Gynecol. 2008;32(1):82–6.

Index

A
Acoustic shadowing, 10–11
Adenomyosis, 97
Aliasing, 22–24
Ano-rectal ultrasound
  adenocarcinoma, 121, 122
  end-fire transducer, 121, 122
  transrectal guided core biopsy, 121, 123
Attenuation, 5–6

B
Backscatter, 17, 18
Beam steering, 17
Bioultrasonics
  attenuation, 5–6
  impedance, 8–9
  reflection, 7–8
  refraction, 6

C
Chronic anal pain
  rectal carcinoma, 139, 140
  squamous cell carcinoma, 139
  trans-spincteric abscess, 138, 139
Chronic pelvic pain syndrome (CPPS), 51–52
Color Doppler, 15–17
  with spectral display, 18, 19
Corpus luteal cyst, 101, 102
CPPS. *See* Chronic pelvic pain syndrome (CPPS)
Cystocele, 141–142

D
Diffuse reflection, 7
Doppler effect, 13–14
Doppler ultrasound, 13
  aliasing, 22–24
  twinkle artifact, 21–22

E
Edging artifact, 11
Endoanal ultrasound
  ano-rectal tumours
    adenocarcinoma, 121, 122
    end-fire transducer, 121, 122
    transrectal guided core biopsy, 121, 123
  indications, 109
  perianal pain and sepsis
    horseshoe abscess, 117, 118
    intersphincteric abscess, 119
    posterior abscess cavity, 117, 118
    retrorectal abscess, 119, 120
    trans-sphincteric fistula, 115–117
  sphincter, 111, 112
    ano-vaginal fistula, 114
    anterior external defect, 114
    distal anal canal, 111, 113
    mid anal canal, 111, 113
    rectal prolapse, 114, 116
    surgical treatment, 114–116
    upper anal canal, 111, 112
  3D endoanal transducer, 109–111
  2D transducer, 109, 110
Endometrial carcinoma, 98, 100
Endometrial hyperplasia, 98, 100

L. Chan et al. (eds.), *Pelvic Floor Ultrasound: Principles, Applications and Case Studies*, DOI 10.1007/978-3-319-04310-4

Endometrial polyps, 97–99
Endometrioma, 102–104

F
Female pelvic organs
  adenomyosis, 97
  corpus luteal cyst, 101, 102
  endometrioma, 102–104
  endometrium, 93
  hydrosalpinx, 105–106
  intramural fibroid, 95–96
  IUCD
    carcinoma, 98, 100
    hyperplasia, 98, 100
    polyps, 97–99
  Nabothian follicle, 91–92
  ovarian cyst, 99, 101
  pathologies, 93, 94
  polycystic ovary, 102, 103
  postmenopausal ovary, 93, 94
  solid ovarian tumour, 104–105
  submucous fibroids, 96
  transabdominal imaging, 87, 88
    left adnexa/ovary, 88, 89
    mid-sagittal plane, 88, 89
    pelvic mass, 88
  transvaginal imaging, 87, 88, 90–91
Female voiding dysfunction
  dynamic imaging, 68–69
  neurogenic bladder dysfunction, 74–75
  persisting incontinence post sling procedure, 70–72
  recurrent urinary infections, 72–73
  severe urinary incontinence, 70, 71
  stress urinary incontinence, 69, 70
  transabdominal ultrasound, 63, 64
  transperineal ultrasound
    imaging, 68, 69
    transducer placement, 63, 65
    2D imaging, 67–68
  video urodynamics, 66–67
  voiding dysfunction post sling procedure, 74

G
Gray-scale ultrasound, 13

H
Harmonic scanning, 20
Hydrosalpinx, 105–106

I
Image optimization techniques
  interfaces, 26–28
  monitor display, 28–29
  orientation, 29
  transducer selection, 25–27
  user-controlled variables
    acoustic output, 30–31
    axial resolution, 32–34
    cine function, 36–37
    depth/size function, 36, 37
    field of view, 36, 37
    focal zone adjustments, 34–36
    frequency, 32–34
    gain, 29–31
    lateral resolution, 34–35
    TGC, 31–32
Impedance, 8–9
Intramural fibroid, 95–96
Intrauterine contraceptive device (IUCD)
  carcinoma, 98, 100
  hyperplasia, 98, 100
  polyps, 97–99
Intrinsic urethral sphincter deficiency (ISD), 70, 71
IUCD. *See* Intrauterine contraceptive device (IUCD)

L
Levator avulsion (LA), 142–144

M
Male voiding dysfunction
  intravesical prostatic protrusion
    bladder calculus, 53, 54
    bladder diverticulum, 53, 54
    bladder outlet obstruction, 53, 55
    imaging protocol, 53, 56
    reduced detrusor compliance, 53, 55
    trabeculation of bladder wall, 53
  physiotherapy management
    CPPS, 51–52
    SUI, 50–51
  post prostatectomy incontinence, 57, 58
    pressure regulating balloon, 57, 59
    scanning techniques, 50, 57
  post prostatectomy incontinence (failed male sling)
    AdVance sling at rest, 59, 60
    re-do AdVance XP sling, 59, 61
    scanning technique, 50, 59
    transobturator slings, 59

transabdominal ultrasound
intravesical prostatic protrusion measurement, 46, 48
of pelvis, 45, 46
postvoid residual urine volume measurement, 46, 47
prostate volume measurement, 46, 48
pubic symphysis, 46, 47
scanning techniques, 46, 49
transperineal ultrasound
scanning technique, 50
transducer placement, 49
Multi planar reconstruction (MPR), 127–128, 130–132

N

Nabothian follicle, 91–92
Neurogenic bladder dysfunction, 74–75

O

Ovarian cyst, 99, 101

P

Pelvic organ prolapse (POP)
anatomy of, 77, 78
coronal reconstruction, 142, 143
cystocele, 141–142
levator avulsion, 142–144
3D/4D pelvic floor ultrasound
rectocele, 84
with recurrent pop, 82–84
symptomatic Pop-Q stage 3 cystocel, 81–82
transperineal imaging technique of, 79–81
ultrasonic disposition, 77, 79
ultrasound, assessment of, 78
Perianal pain and sepsis
horseshoe abscess, 117, 118
intersphincteric abscess, 119
posterior abscess cavity, 117, 118
retrorectal abscess, 119, 120
trans-sphincteric fistula, 115–117
Persistent incontinence post sling, 70–72
Piezoelectric effect, 1–2
Polycystic ovary, 102, 103
POP. *See* Pelvic organ prolapse (POP)
POP-Q Quantification System, 82, 83
Post prostatectomy incontinence, 57, 58
failed male sling
AdVance sling at rest, 59, 60
re-do AdVance XP sling, 59, 61
scanning technique, 50, 59
transobturator slings, 59
pressure regulating balloon, 57, 59
scanning techniques, 50, 57
Power Doppler ultrasonography, 17–18
PRF. *See* Pulse repetition frequency (PRF)
Pulsed-wave ultrasound, 3, 4
Pulse repetition frequency (PRF), 3

R

Recurrent urinary infections, 72–73
Reflection, 7–8
Refraction, 6
Region of interest (ROI), 128, 129
Resistive index (RI), 18, 19
Reverberation artifact, 12–13

S

Severe urinary incontinence, 70, 71
Solid ovarian tumour, 104–105
Spatial compounding, 20, 21
Speckle effect, 7
Spectral Doppler, 22, 23
Spectral waveform, 18, 19
Specular reflection, 7
Sphincter, 111, 112
ano-vaginal fistula, 114
anterior external defect, 114
distal anal canal, 111, 113
mid anal canal, 111, 113
rectal prolapse, 114, 116
surgical treatment, 114–116
upper anal canal, 111, 112
Stress urinary incontinence (SUI), 50–51, 69, 70
Submucous fibroids, 96
SUI. *See* Stress urinary incontinence (SUI)

T

TGC. *See* Time-gain compensation (TGC)
3D/4D pelvic floor ultrasound
rectocele, 84
with recurrent pop, 82–84
symptomatic Pop-Q stage 3 cystocel, 81–82
3D pelvic floor ultrasound
chronic anal pain
rectal carcinoma, 139, 140

3D pelvic floor ultrasound (*cont.*)
squamous cell carcinoma, 139
trans-spincteric abscess, 138, 139
data set
coronal image manipulation, 133
MPR, 130–132
transperineal ultrasound, 130, 131
Macroplastique® bulking agent, 137, 138
POP
coronal reconstruction, 142, 143
cystocele, 141–142
levator avulsion, 142–144
potential applications, 125
2 sling procedures, 136
voiding dysfunction, 133–135
volume acquisition
cross hair, 128
'4D' capability, 126
MPR, 127–128
pixel, 126
ROI, 128, 129
sweep angle, 128, 129
techniques, 129–130
trim line, 128, 129
volume acquisition, 126
voxel, 127
Time-gain compensation (TGC), 31–32
Transabdominal ultrasound
female voiding dysfunction, 63, 64
intravesical prostatic protrusion measurement, 46, 48
of pelvis, 45, 46
postvoid residual urine volume measurement, 46, 47
prostate volume measurement, 46, 48
pubic symphysis, 46, 47
scanning techniques, 46, 49
Transducers, 25–27
Transperineal ultrasound
dynamic imaging, 68, 69
scanning technique, 50
transducer placement, 49, 63, 65
2D imaging, 67–68
Twinkle artifact, 21–22

U

Ultrasound
artifacts associated with Doppler ultrasound
aliasing, 22–24
twinkle artifact, 21–22
assessment of POP, 78–79
common artifacts
acoustic shadowing, 10–11
edging artifact, 11
increased through-transmission, 9–10
reverberation artifact, 12–13
harmonic scanning, 20
interactions with human tissue
attenuation, 5–6
impedance, 8–9
reflection, 7
refraction, 6
modes of
color Doppler, 15–17
Doppler effect, 13–15
Doppler ultrasound, 13
gray-scale ultrasound, 13
power Doppler, 17–18
spectral waveform, 18, 19
physics of
image sequence, 4–5
longitudinal waves, 2, 3
piezoelectric effect, 1–2
pulsed-wave ultrasound, 3, 4
sine wave, 2, 3
velocity, 4
spatial compounding, 20–21
Ultrasound machine settings. *See* Image optimization techniques
Ultrasound ranging, 3, 4
Ultrasound scan setup
equipment selection, 39
equipment setup, maintainence and protection, 40, 41
portable units *vs.* trolley/cart based systems, 39
procedures and accreditation, 42–43
room setup, 40, 42, 43
transducer selection, 40
Urethral hypermobility, 69, 70
Urodynamics, 66–67

V

Video urodynamics, 66–67
Voiding dysfunction post sling, 74